Cancer
Up the
Wazoo

Stories, information, and hope
for those affected by anal cancer

Angela G. Gentile,
Editor and Contributor

Care to Age

Cancer Up the Wazoo:
Stories, information, and hope
for those affected by anal cancer

Copyright © 2018 Angela G. Gentile

The information provided in this book is for educational and entertainment purposes only and is not intended to replace the advice of your doctor, healthcare professional, financial advisor or lawyer. You are encouraged to discuss any concerns you have with a qualified professional.

First Edition
ISBN-13: 978-1986326391
ISBN-10: 198632639X

Care to Age Press. Printed in the USA.

Cancer is a word, not a sentence.

John Diamond

I dedicate this book to all who have been affected by anal cancer: those who were diagnosed and treated for it; the family members and caregivers who suffer along; and the advocates, researchers, and professionals who work tirelessly to ensure the safety and well-being of those they serve. And most importantly—the late Farrah Fawcett for sharing her diagnosis with her fans and bringing forth an awareness of anal cancer.

****

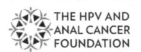

$1.00 (CAD) for every new paperback copy of *Cancer Up the Wazoo* sold will be donated to *The HPV and Anal Cancer Foundation*. The donation will be used in the USA (and UK) to further the Foundation's scientific research funding, programs for thrivers, and vaccine advocacy.

Acknowledgements

Thank you to everyone who contributed to the production of this book. I couldn't have done it without you!

For those who have taken the time to review and edit a chapter, offer suggestions, help with graphics, and correct my typos and grammar, I thank you from the bottom my heart. These special people include: Peggy Belton, Tammy Crumpston, Joan Ellis, Lorenzo Gentile, Marta Grande, Penny Lansdale, Joana Dougherty McGee, Patricia McKinney, Cory Tucker, Pamela Williams, and Virginia Davis Wilson.

I am very grateful for those who have shared their stories and insight, no matter how big or small, including those not on the contributor listing: Dr. Foster Lasley, Dr. Anne Katz, Lynda Sie Greaves, Maureen Warren, Cindy Ring, Carol Anne Hollen, Corrie Yelland, Penny, and Cathy.

A special thank you goes out to Virginia Lloyd-Davies for allowing me to use her Dragonfly and Lotus Chinese Brush Painting artwork. She is a very talented artist—check her out on YouTube!

To my family and friends, especially Agapito (a.k.a. Cupp), Lorenzo, Simone, my mom Virginia Davis Wilson, and my very good friend Sheila Roy, thank you for your unlimited support, love and patience while I wrote, edited, and researched for this book.

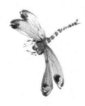

Contents

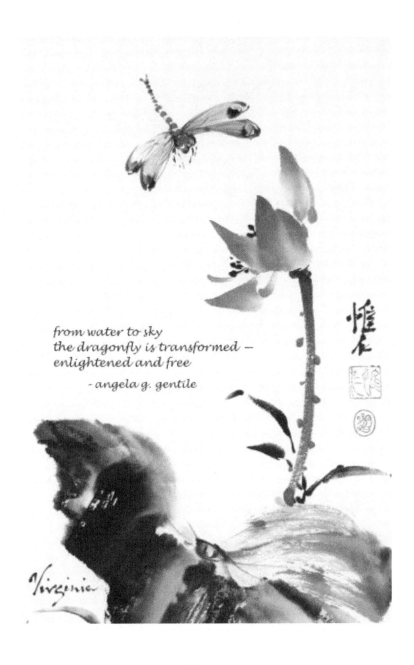

from water to sky
the dragonfly is transformed —
enlightened and free

- angela g. gentile

Introduction

"To know the road ahead, ask those coming back."
–Chinese Proverb

When I was diagnosed with anal cancer in 2017, there was limited knowledge available as it is a rare form of cancer. What I was about to endure was one of the most horrific, brutal, and barbaric cancer treatments. Pelvic radiation therapy, directed toward the tumor in the anal canal, resulted in what I'd call collateral damage. This included radiation burns to the private areas down below. There are many sensitive and delicate body parts and nerves down there. Enduring, healing, and recovering from this kind of ordeal can be very difficult. For others, the experience may not be as traumatic.

My idea for this book came shortly after I finished my chemotherapy and radiation treatment. I was given the "all clear," yet I was not well enough to go back to full-time work. So I did what I love: I came up with an idea to write a book. This book was going to be different. I wanted to give a voice to those who had a story to tell. There were other books written about anal cancer, but many were written by women from their own perspectives. I wanted to create a book that included a diverse and broad range of experiences and voices, one that would help the newly diagnosed, their loved ones, and the professionals. It wasn't a difficult decision to make. I wanted to produce an anthology, a collection of true stories. Chapters would be inspired by experiences. Basically, I wanted to write the book I would have wanted to read when I was newly diagnosed.

What you are about to read is based on true stories, stories of men and women who have been affected by cancer. There are voices of mothers, friends, and professionals–all sharing their stories. Some stories and passages will touch your heart. Some will make you laugh. You may find yourself inspired and full of hope. You will read about the fears, anxieties, and other difficulties we go through as we plod along this so-called journey of cancer. Unexpected blessings and lessons learned will also be shared.

We can't possibly cover all the issues that will come up with anal cancer and its treatment, so we offer our own stories. This is what we know. Some of the chapters are based on what we feel you need to know as a newly diagnosed patient. Those new to the world of anal cancer will find helpful information in the chapter on the basics. We've tried to hit on all the most common themes and topics we've come across in our experiences.

Your experience will be similar but different than ours. I hope you can use this book as a reference, referring to it during your cancer treatment and recovery journey. Share relevant chapters with friends, family, and professionals so they can understand more about what you are going through and how they can best help you.

Some writers use explicit imagery and language, so consider yourself forewarned! Don't let the "F-word" scare you! Also—some stories are graphic and may shock some readers.

Whether you believe in God, a higher power, Creator, source, or nothing, you will get something out of this book. It just so happens many of the writers (myself included) are Christian. Our illness has heightened our spiritual connectedness in many cases. If that is not your belief, I respect that.

I've made a concerted effort to produce a collection that is helpful, insightful, hopeful, and full of resources, tips, and ideas. The index in the back will help you find whatever it is you are looking for, whether it's to review something you've already read, or to go straight to the topic you are most interested in. I've included references as appropriate at the end of each chapter. A glossary will help you understand terms you may not be familiar with. There are other resources and helpful sections that will provide you with the necessary guidance you may require. I hesitated to put website links, as I know sometimes these links disappear or get broken—but it is a risk I was willing to take.

And on that note, if you find any erroneous information or broken links, or if you think of something that should be included in a revised edition, please contact me at caretoage@gmail.com.

Disclaimer: The information provided in this book is for educational and entertainment purposes only and is not intended to replace the advice of your doctor, healthcare professional, financial advisor or lawyer. You are encouraged to discuss any concerns you have with a qualified professional.

Warm regards,

Angela G. Gentile

Chapter 1

Anal Cancer Basics

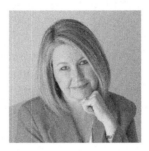

Angela G. Gentile

The word "cancer," or the term "Big C" as some of us know it, is all too familiar. Most of us learn at a very young age how cancer can rob us of our relatives, friends, neighbors or acquaintances. We hear about it on the news, how cancer is something to be "fought" and "prevented." Cancer is one of the leading causes of death in North America, with one in every three women and one in every two men affected. One in two Canadians will develop cancer in their lifetime, and one in four will die from it. Not all types of cancer are fatal, and the good news is that people who are diagnosed with cancer are living longer thanks to modern-day medicine.

Cancer is an umbrella term used to describe over 100 types of diseases that cause the body's healthy cells to develop into abnormal cells which can grow and spread. These tumors, blood, or bone diseases can cause other problems, and some eventually spread throughout the body or "metastasize." When cancer metastasizes, it is challenging to treat. When vital organs such as the lungs or liver are affected it becomes life-threatening.

Everyone is at risk of developing cancer, even people who live a healthy lifestyle and avoid risk factors such as smoking, drinking alcohol, and inhaling toxins like asbestos. Researchers are learning more about cancer and its causes, but unfortunately, no one is immune. Every age, race and gender can develop cancer; however, in Canada, 89% of those diagnosed with cancer are 50 and older. The longer we live, the more chances we have of developing life-threatening illnesses such as cancer and heart disease. There is no cancer cure-all, but fortunately we have some very effective treatments to keep it in check.

The most commonly diagnosed forms of cancer in those 50 and older are lung, colorectal, breast (in women), and prostate (in men). Lung cancer is the leading cause of cancer deaths in both men and women. People who smoke are at high risk for lung cancer.

Anal Cancer is Rare

Although rare, anal cancer is on the rise—especially in women aged 50-69 (Van Dyne et al., 2018). The reason for the increasing rate of anal cancer is not fully known (Ahmedin et. al, 2013). In 2013, 580 Canadians were diagnosed with anal cancer. The American Cancer Society estimates there will be about 8,580 Americans diagnosed with anal cancer in 2018. About 65% of these new cases will be in women, with the average age at diagnosis being in the early 60s. Our lifetime risk of developing anal cancer is estimated at 1 in 500 people (versus 1 in 9 for breast cancer and 1 in 11 for lung cancer).

Experts agree that human papillomavirus (HPV) infections are linked to the development of certain cancers such as anal, cervical, sexual organs, mouth, and throat. The HPV and Anal Cancer Foundation states, "Nearly all sexually active adults will have at least one type of sexually transmitted HPV at some point in their lifetime. It can be transmitted through skin-to-skin contact during sexual activity. HPV can be spread without engaging in sexual intercourse" (HPV: The Facts). It is estimated that HPV causes 93% of anal cancer.

Anal cancer affects the gastrointestinal tract and is often mistaken for rectal cancer. The anal canal is the lowest part of the colon, located in the area between the rectum and the anus (butt hole). The anal canal houses the anal sphincter muscles, which are responsible for holding back feces (poop) before it leaves the body.

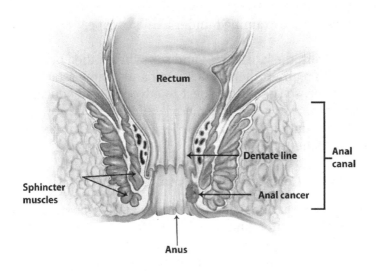

Figure 1. Anal Cancer (Tumor) and Surrounding Anatomy

Growths and abnormal cells can develop in the anal area. People who have anal warts are more likely to be diagnosed with anal cancer. Pre-cancerous conditions called low-grade anal intraepithelial neoplasia (AIN) or high-grade anal squamous intraepithelial lesions (SIL) are also known as dysplasia. High-grade SIL is the more serious of the two and needs to be watched closely.

In anal cancer, a tumor or a malignant (cancerous) lump starts developing in the anal canal. If it is large enough, it may begin to interfere with bowel movements. Growths can also be on the outside of the anus.

There are different types of anal cancer, the most common being "squamous cell carcinoma," which is often (but not always) related to the human papillomavirus (HPV). Cancer can develop 20-30 years after exposure to HPV. HPV is also responsible for other cancers found in the cervix, mouth, throat and neck.

The other types of anal cancers are called cloacogenic carcinoma, adenocarcinoma, basal cell carcinoma and melanoma. The type of cancer cells found in the anal area can be determined by a biopsy, where the cells are examined under a microscope.

Farrah Fawcett, the late actress and sex symbol, died of anal cancer in 2009. She realized there was stigma and shame attached to this type of cancer, so she did her best to advocate and educate others. She shared her story in the media, and there is now a Farrah Fawcett Foundation to honor her legacy. We address stigma and shame throughout this book.

What I Have Learned About Anal Cancer

I have endured treatment and I am a survivor of anal cancer. During my cancer encounter and sharing with others, I learned about symptoms, diagnosis, treatment, and recovering from treatment. Concerned about some of my symptoms, I did what most computer-literate people do—I Googled it. I was experiencing some of the signs of anal cancer, which made my heart sink. I remember the moment I told my daughter, "I think I have anal cancer."

Symptoms of Anal Cancer (American Cancer Society):

- Rectal bleeding

- Rectal itching

- A lump or mass at the anal opening

- Pain or a feeling of fullness in the anal area

- Narrowing of the stool or other changes in bowel movements

- Abnormal discharge from the anus

- Swollen lymph nodes in the anal or groin areas

Some people experience no symptoms. Often, symptoms are misdiagnosed as hemorrhoids, even by doctors. Anal fissures, fistulas, abscesses, and anal warts can also be causes for some of these symptoms, so it is vital to get assessed by a doctor.

Diagnosing Anal Cancer

Diagnosing anal cancer can be done in a few ways. For me, the digital rectal exam (DRE) helped with the diagnosis. A DRE is a simple procedure that can be done at the doctor's office. The doctor inserts a lubricated, gloved finger into the anus, and feels for any abnormalities or blood. If a lump or blood is found, the doctor can order or perform more tests, such as a colonoscopy, endoscopy, anoscopy, CT scan, MRI, PET scan, and biopsy (as mentioned previously). I had everything except the endoscopy and anoscopy. Blood tests, urine tests, and physical examination of the abdomen and surrounding areas are also usually performed. Sometimes an anal or vaginal Pap test is also done (a small sample of cells are removed and examined under a microscope). The rigid proctosigmoidoscope (defined as a thin, lighted instrument to examine the rectum and lower part of the colon) is also something that may be used to help the doctor see the insides of the lower part of the colon, rectum, and anal canal.

Based on all the tests and exams, the doctor will know what kind of cancer it is and what stage it is. There are four stages of any cancer diagnosis. The stages are dependent on the size and spread of cancer. Stage 1 cancer is early, and stage 4 is when cancer has grown and spread throughout the body. I was diagnosed with squamous cell carcinoma of the anal canal, stage 3, as I had one affected lymph node.

Anal cancer rarely spreads (metastasizes) to distant organs in the body, but when it does, it usually affects the liver or the lungs. The spread is generally through the blood supply, tissues, or lymph system. (This is what happened to Farrah Fawcett.)

The medical exam will also include some medical history. The specialist (for me, it was a colorectal surgeon) will want to know more about your overall health and medical history in order to make some decisions about how to treat the cancer. There may also be a need for a second opinion, as some people need that reassurance. A doctor or a person with cancer can request a second opinion.

What Are the Risks Associated with Anal Cancer

Many people who have not heard or read about anal cancer may want to know how they got it. Mayo Clinic has listed lifestyle and other risk factors linked to anal cancer:

Who is at Risk for Anal Cancer:

- Those 50 and older.
- Those having had four or more sexual partners over a lifetime (increases HPV infection risk).
- Those who engage in anal sex, especially receptive anal sex (men who have sex with men are at high risk).
- Smokers may be at increased risk of anal cancer.
- Those with a history of cancer. Women who have had cervical, vulvar, or vaginal cancer have an increased risk.
- Those infected with the human papillomavirus (HPV). This sexually transmitted infection, which causes genital (including anal) warts can also cause anal cancer.
- Those who have used drugs or have conditions that suppress your immune system. Transplant patients or people with human immunodeficiency virus (HIV)—the virus that causes acquired immune deficiency syndrome (AIDS)—have an increased risk of anal cancer.

Although it's an embarrassing area to show the doctor, warts in the genital and anal areas should be assessed, and preferably removed (they can be "burnt off" in the doctor's office).

Here is a note about HPV getting into the anal canal. Women are taught to wipe from front to back. My gynecologist tells me HPV can be spread to the anus and surrounding area by performing this common daily habit (Ladies—dab, don't wipe!).

The colorectal surgeon also said that many people are infected with HPV, and they never go on to develop cancer. Additionally, HPV can be transferred from mother to baby during childbirth.

I also wonder if there is a genetic component to this, as my grandmother was diagnosed with vulvar cancer in her later years.

How Can Anal Cancer Be Prevented—It Can't Be, *Butt* . . .

Mayo Clinic's website also states there is "no sure way" to prevent anal cancer. There are ways to reduce the risk, however, including the following:

- Practice safer sex. For those who want to reduce their risk of anal cancer—abstaining from sex, using a condom during sex, using a condom or dental/oral dam during oral sex—can help protect against HPV or HIV infection. Both increase your risk for anal cancer.

- Stop smoking. Smoking increases your risk of anal cancer. Don't start smoking, and quit if you currently do. Doctors have solutions to help you kick the habit.

- Prevent via vaccination against HPV. There are currently two vaccines on the market that are given to boys and girls. Speak to your child's healthcare team about this vaccine. Younger adults are also encouraged to get the vaccine, up until their early twenties.

- HPV vaccination may help reduce the risk of anal cancer recurrence. The research is ongoing in this area as it is fairly new. The results for men have been promising. (As an aside, I have been vaccinated after treatment, after much encouragement from my gynecologist and family doctor.)

Early Detection is Your Best Bet

Early detection measures are strongly recommended for anyone who falls into the risk categories. This may mean a regular anal Pap test, a digital rectal exam, a colonoscopy, and investigation of any abnormal or painful symptoms in the anal area. I would suggest that if you suspect it's more than a hemorrhoid, request more tests until the doctor has been able to rule out anal cancer. Unfortunately, hemorrhoids are a very common initial misdiagnosis which allows for more time to pass without prompt, critical treatment. Insist on further investigations such as a biopsy or rigid proctoscope examination.

At times someone may be diagnosed with "precancerous" cells as well as dysplasia. Anal precancer, or "anal intraepithelial neoplasia," has its own kind of treatment such as laser ablation or topical chemotherapy. Polyps (clumps of often abnormal cells) in the colon are also found to be linked to cancer. Regular follow up and treatment, as recommended by your doctor, can help prevent the growth, development, and spread of cancer.

Treating Anal Cancer

Average prognosis (likely outcome of the disease and its treatment) for someone diagnosed with anal cancer is about a 67% chance of survival for five years. After five years, close monitoring is usually not required. Treatment usually consists of a combination of radiation and chemotherapy. Surgery (removing the tumor) is often not the first option for treatment.

The Canadian Cancer Society defines radiation therapy as high doses of radiation (energy moving through space) used to destroy cancer cells, slow down cell growth, and shrink tumors. Daily treatments damage the cancer cells over and over again. The cancer cells don't have a chance to repair themselves between treatments, so eventually, they die.

Chemotherapy is a drug therapy used to destroy cancer cells or slow their growth. It can be in liquid form (given intravenously) or in pill form (taken by mouth). Also known as chemo, it is often given in combination with other anticancer drugs or agents.

The "Nigro Protocol" is the most common and successful treatment for the majority of anal cancer cases. It consists of 30 days of pelvic radiation, with the targets being the tumor and lymph nodes, if present, and two rounds of chemotherapy. For me, it was mitomycin (a.k.a. Mitomycin-C) and fluorouracil, commonly known as "5-FU." There are variations of this protocol; some have more or fewer radiation treatments and different types of chemotherapy. This treatment has been used since the 1970s, as a better or more successful treatment plan has yet to be discovered.

The surgeon explained chemotherapy "sensitizes" the tumor and helps the radiation do its job more efficiently by shrinking or destroying the tumor. In addition to the intravenous chemotherapy treatments, there will be a number of blood tests, so many opt to have a peripherally inserted central catheter (PICC), which is a semi-permanent opening for injections and other needle procedures, inserted into the arm. Alternatively, one may get an implanted central vascular access device (CVAD) or port, which is a long tube placed in a large vein in the upper chest, under the skin. A catheter, or small tube, connects the port to the vein.

Unfortunately, radiation to the pelvic region is perhaps the most brutal of all cancer treatments, but it is also very effective. Dr. Foster Lasley, a radiation oncologist, states, "Anal cancer is different from other types of pelvic radiation because I am radiating so low and hitting very sensitive areas that have rich innervation. I would probably agree with anal carcinoma being probably the most brutal thing I do in terms of acute side effects. On a scale of 1-10, I'd give it a 9.5. I reserve 10 for those wacky, terrible cases I see sometimes."

> TIP: The National Comprehensive Cancer Network has a thorough "Clinical Practice Guidelines" for Anal Carcinoma, found at (Login required):
> www.nccn.org/professionals/physician_gls/PDF/anal.pdf.

Your Team

The person with anal cancer will need an oncology or healthcare team of professionals working together to optimize treatment and keep side effects to a minimum. Side-effect management is essential, and many people will experience radiation burns to the pelvic area (including anal, perianal, genitals, groin), and will require pain management, skin treatments, and other symptom management.

Team members may include the radiation oncologist and nurse, the radiation team, the chemotherapy doctor (medical oncologist), colorectal surgeon, your family doctor, the on-call weekend and evening team, social worker, dietician and more! You may also consider having a psychologist or psychiatrist help you with emotional and mood problems if they arise.

> A support group is a group of people with similar disease or concerns who help each other cope by sharing experiences and information.
> —National Cancer Institute

Your supports (practical, emotional, and informational) will hopefully include family members, friends, support groups (whether in-person or online), and other people diagnosed with cancer.

Side Effects of Treatment

Anal cancer treatment (radiation, chemotherapy, and sometimes surgery) usually takes about six weeks from start to finish. There are numerous side effects to watch for, some being very serious.

Neutropenia is very common in people being treated for cancer, as chemotherapy depletes the immune system, which consists of white blood cells. White blood cells help the body protect against infections and foreign invaders. Neutropenia is a life-threatening condition determined through a blood test and can come on very suddenly. When the person becomes neutropenic, physicians address the issue. Check out *chemocare.com* for more info on side effects of chemotherapy.

It is critical for someone diagnosed with neutropenia to not expose oneself to anything that could cause an infection, as the body cannot fight it. For example, I was advised to postpone my visit to the dentist when my white blood cell count was low.

Severe fatigue (tiredness) often comes with radiation. This fatigue can impact a person even when radiation is used to treat a small area of skin cancer on the tip of someone's nose. However,

Dr. Foster Lasley, a radiation oncologist, states there isn't a reasonable biological explanation for this. He tells his patients to stay as active as possible, and post-treatment, he expects people to feel about 50% better after one month and 80% better by three months. It may take up to a full year before they are back to their prior energy level. He adds that anal cancer is particularly brutal when it comes to some other side effects, so that timeline is sometimes skewed a little further out. This fatigue can also affect one's mood, and although it doesn't cause depression, it can certainly make it worse. If fatigue is an issue, it's always important to talk to the medical team, as there could be other explanations for it.

Side effects vary, and there is quite a range. For example, I know of some people who hardly missed a day of work. Some have minimal side effects. While others lose their hair, my hair thinned. I remember having "chemo brain" or "chemo fog"—a very common state of distraction, or not being quite "with it" while on chemotherapy. For example, I couldn't remember which finger I wore my wedding ring on—was it the right or left hand?

A full list of radiation or chemotherapy side effects can be obtained from your healthcare team. The pharmacist gave me an excellent overview of the chemotherapy I was receiving, and the radiation team gave me some handouts on pelvic radiation side effects to watch for (like losing your pubic hair!). The pharmacist warned me about mouth sores as a side effect of chemotherapy, too.

Recovering and Healing After Treatment for Anal Cancer

Although the treatment is completed in about six weeks, often there is a lengthy recovery process. Depending on each person's response to radiation and chemotherapy, people who work may need to take some time off. It may take up to a year to feel ready to go back to work. In the short term, responsibilities may need to be delegated to others. There are psychological and physical changes that can affect a person's outlook, priorities, and mood.

During and after treatment, it's important to do as much as you can and get moving. It can help reverse some downward momentum—

even if it's just walking to the mailbox or pushing a shopping cart for support.

There may be unexpected things that happen. I experienced "stranding" and fibrous tissue in the anal canal and vaginal walls. Fat stranding is best described as folds of fat that are thickened and inflamed due to radiation injury. I also experienced vaginal stenosis (narrowing of the vagina). It is suggested that ALL women who have pelvic radiation use a vaginal dilator daily to PREVENT vaginal narrowing or stenosis. Stiff hips and groin can also result. There can be unexpected injuries or trauma, also known as "collateral damage," to the surrounding organs and skin tissues. Some end up with pelvic radiation disease also known as radiation-induced injury (interestingly, pelvic radiation disease is not commonly recognized in the USA). Pelvic floor physiotherapy can help with improving some of the after-effects of radiation. Treatment can make a woman go into menopause. I've heard it said that radiation to the pelvis is like putting your private parts and organs into a microwave oven. It all gets fried. But this is what is needed to destroy the cancer cells.

There are ways to combat and heal from many, but not all of these after-effects. It takes time, patience, commitment, and work. Late effects can also happen, as radiation has come to be known as "the gift that keeps on giving." For example, if lymph nodes in the groin have been zapped, lymphedema, or swelling of the legs can occur even years later.

Exploring Alternative Options

When I was diagnosed, I also explored other treatment options. I read about alternative medicine, but I was not convinced there was a better way to go. One woman shared her story about a cannabis oil (marijuana) cure for her anal cancer. After I did some research, I was not convinced it would treat my condition, so I stuck with the original plan. I had a friend look into alternatives for me, but she couldn't come up with anything else. I asked a Facebook friend to connect me with someone who took the natural route as she "knew so many." She never got back to me.

There are many alternative remedies for pain relief, including cannabis, Chinese herbs, natural supplements, etc. Also, many have found relief from TENS (Transcutaneous Electrical Nerve Stimulation) units, which run a non-painful, mild electric current through electrodes placed on the skin. Home remedies such as warm baths in baking soda and essential oils can offer comfort. Meditation, massage, and chiropractic adjustments can also provide some people relief. (More on this in a later chapter on Integrative Medicine.)

Abdominoperineal Resection with Permanent Colostomy

One option for those who have no success with chemoradiation treatment (or for those with the melanoma or adenocarcinoma type of cancer) is to have surgery to remove the tumor. The tumor could be removed if it is suitable for this type of operation. If the mass is large or has grown deeper into the tissues, a more intensive surgery called abdominoperineal resection (APR) may be required. If the sphincter muscles don't work correctly (a loss of controlling bowel function, for example) or the tumor compromises the anus, this is an option. It results in a permanent colostomy. (Colostomies can also be temporary if the doctor deems it a necessary procedure to manage pain or other problems with functioning.)

With APR surgery, the anus is closed up (a.k.a. "Barbie butt") and a colostomy is necessary. A colostomy is a permanent hole made in the abdomen. The colon is connected to it, and the feces (poop) is emptied into a bag outside of the body instead of through the anus. The vast majority of those who have had these procedures report that after a period of adjustment (diet/maintenance/emotions), they live very active, healthy, happy lives.

Clinical Trials May Be Available

Another option for people who don't respond to the standard treatment for anal cancer, or who have an advanced form of cancer, is to explore the possibility of clinical trials. Participating in a clinical trial is a way to help researchers test the effectiveness of new treatments and drugs. People volunteer for these studies and report on the efficacy of the treatment and any side effects. Dr. Cathy Eng, who is a Gastrointestinal Oncologist at the MD Anderson Cancer

Center in Texas, USA, has been the principal investigator in some of these studies. For example, immunotherapy (prevention or treatment of disease using substances that stimulate the body's immune response) is an emerging science in the area of cancer treatment. There are always new treatments being developed and tested, so you can ask your doctor about clinical trials you may be considered for. You can also check online at *ClinicalTrials.gov*.

The Integrated Cancer Care Approach is Best (in my opinion)

I highly recommend hospitals or cancer centers that promote and encourage an integrated approach to care. These are centers with clinicians, doctors, and specialists practicing orthodox or allopathic (traditional) medicine who are also open to helping a patient decide on complementary therapies that may help, such as massage, yoga, meditation, prayer, and support groups. Those who do not have access to such centers can create networks to benefit from an integrated program.

For some people, acupuncture has helped relieve the symptoms of nausea associated with cancer treatment. Unfortunately, many complementary and alternative therapies lack scientific proof of effectiveness. Others prove to be no more helpful than a placebo. A placebo effect means relief has been brought about not by a medicinal reaction, but by the person imagining it is going to work—relief resulting from the brain "convincing the body." I am of the mindset that if it doesn't harm, and it doesn't interfere with standard treatment, and it's not breaking the bank, it's worth a try. If the service or product comes with a money-back guarantee, that's even better! Some of these integrated centers offer a variety of programs for free as part of their comprehensive care approach. I believe the body-mind-spirit approach is necessary to help one through a traumatic and life-threatening cancer ordeal. (More on the integrative approach in a later chapter.)

Post-Treatment Follow Up and Monitoring

Once treatment ends, and there is an "all clear," "no evidence of disease (NED)" or "cancer-free" declaration by the specialist, a follow-up plan is made. You will be seen by a surgeon, a radiation

> I may be disease-free, but I am not free
> from my disease. –Angela G. Gentile

oncologist, a medical oncologist, or other specialist for regular monitoring for a specified amount of time, which could be years. These regular visits, which could be every three months, six months, or something along those lines can cause people anxiety and fear of recurrence. Waiting for the results of tests such as CT scans can cause "scanxiety" for some. The anxiety caused by the time it takes to wait for results can create fear of an abnormal result.

On my initial six-month follow-up exam, the doctor stated he saw "No Evidence of Recurrent Disease." I jokingly and happily announced, "So I am a NERD!" (I've also since heard NERD can mean "No Evidence of Residual Disease.")

Finding a "New Normal"

An anal cancer diagnosis is not a death sentence. It can be overcome with early detection, proper diagnosis, standard treatment combined with complementary or integrated approaches, and a team of professionals and other supports. Participating in cancer rehabilitation programs, which may include exercise, yoga, support, etc.; planning a trip; or getting a puppy are examples of things that can help you move forward. Most people say they must find a "new normal" after a cancer diagnosis, as it often has a profound way of changing a person's mental attitude, outlook, and priorities. Some people retire, change jobs, or find an entirely new purpose in helping others who have also experienced cancer. Living well with or after cancer takes some effort. You can do it.

****

REFERENCES:

Ahmedin, J., Simard, E. P., Dorell, C., Noone, A., Markowitz., L. E., Kohler, B., Eheman, C., Saraiya, M., Bandi, P., Saslow, D., Cronin, K. A., Watson, M., Schiffman, M., Henley, S., J., Schymura, M. J., Anderson, R. N., Yankey, D., & Edwards, B. K., (2013). Annual Report to the Nation on the Status of

Cancer, 1975-2009, Featuring the Burden and Trends in Human Papillomavirus (HPV)-Associated Cancers and HPV Vaccination Coverage Levels. *Journal of the National Cancer Institute*, 105(3): 175-201. doi: 10.1093/jnci/djs491

Van Dyne, E. A., Henley, S. J., Saraiya, M., Thomas, C. C., Markowitz, L. E. Benard, V. B. (2018). Trends in Human Papillomavirus-Associated Cancers—United States, 1999-2015. *Morbidity and Mortality Weekly Report of CDC*, 24 Aug 2018, 67(33): 918-924. Retrieved 26 Aug 2018.

RESOURCES:

American Cancer Society (*cancer.org*)

Canadian Cancer Society (*cancer.ca)*

Centers for Disease Control and Prevention (*cdc.gov*)

ChemoCare (*chemocare.com*)

The Farrah Fawcett Foundation (*thefarrahfawcettfoundation.org)*

The HPV and Anal Cancer Foundation (*analcancerfoundation.org)*

Mayo Clinic (*mayoclinic.org*)

National Cancer Institute (*cancer.gov)*

National Comprehensive Cancer Network Guidelines for Anal Carcinoma (Login required) (*nccn.org/professionals/physician_gls/PDF/anal.pdf)*

Chapter 2

For the Newly Diagnosed

Angela G. Gentile

"Courage is being scared to death but saddling up anyway."
—John Wayne

"This is all presumptive. We don't have any pathology yet. But I can tell you based on what I saw today, this is cancer. That's what this is."

Those words from the specialist numbed me to the bone. My immediate thoughts were—my kids will be devastated. Will I survive this? Then other thoughts and fears came—my mom will crumble. Will I lose my hair? Will chemo make me sick? Can I afford this? I am being robbed of my old age. I'll never see my grandchildren. I won't get to grow old with my husband.

Being told you have cancer is a shocking and surreal experience. It doesn't matter if you were suspecting it or it came out of the blue, it's still devastating. When I was diagnosed with anal cancer, I was with my husband when the colorectal surgeon told me those words. Although I was suspecting and fearing the worst, it still didn't feel real. The next few days, weeks, and months ahead were one big whirlwind of emotions, medical tests, waiting, treatments, side effects, and so much more. I learned so much during this encounter with cancer.

In this chapter, I will write specifically for those who are newly diagnosed with anal cancer. One of the first things you may want to do is read up on what anal cancer is. There is a lot of information on the Internet, and not all of it is helpful. Ask your doctors for recommendations on trusted resources (such as *cancer.gov*). Contact your local cancer organizations for information on education, meetings, groups, etc. If you haven't read Chapter One in this book on the basics of anal cancer, you may want to do that now. Get those closest to you to read it too.

Hopefully this chapter will help you understand yourself, your situation, your family, and your upcoming cancer ordeal. My intent and wish are that it will help you cope. I hope it encourages you to be gentle and kind to yourself. This Body-Mind-Spirit holistic approach to dealing with cancer and its treatment will help you get through this. Assisting others through a similar experience will also make me feel better, even if I help only one person.

Learning of the Diagnosis

Everyone's cancer is different. Even those who have the same type of cancer soon realize there are various factors involved. What was your health like before diagnosis? Are there complicating factors to your overall health status? What stage (how far along and widespread) is your cancer? How big is your tumor? What kind of cancer cells are they? Where exactly is the cancer located, and what is it affecting? Is there pain? Do you need pain relief? How are your coping skills?

There are many questions to ask and a lot of information to take in when you receive a diagnosis. Sometimes more tests need to be done before the whole situation is known. Sometimes people like to get a second opinion, and sometimes even doctors want a second opinion. As a person newly diagnosed with cancer, these kinds of things may or may not go through your mind. I think it's important to have an explanation of the type of cancer you have and the stage of the disease (there are four stages). Have it written down, so you don't forget. Make copies of scans or other test results. This will be helpful down the road.

Questions you may want to ask your doctor include:

- What kind of cancer do I have?
- How did I get this?

- What are my treatment options?
- What happens if I don't get the treatment?
- What are the side effects?
- Would you do this treatment?

The initial reaction, emotionally, is also very personal. Depending on what you know about cancer, if you've had experiences in your family or social network, this will affect your thoughts and feelings about cancer. Our expectations and what we know of cancer may also be influenced by what we see in movies and on television. What we know now is that this isn't your grandmother's cancer, and anal cancer does not mean a death sentence. Medical therapy and research have come a long way concerning treating cancer, and many people are living with (and after) it.

Treatment decisions will also need to be made. With all the information at hand, your specialist will present the best treatment plan. You may want to ask about things such as side effects, risks, and other options. You want to be optimistic about your treatment, as a positive outlook can significantly improve your coping skills and quality of life as you go through the procedures.

Integrative medicine (complementary treatments as well as conventional medical therapies and treatments) combines the best of both worlds. I would strongly recommend exploring complementary therapies such as massage, yoga, and acupuncture with your cancer team. Mind-body therapies such as yoga and meditation can help foster a positive mindset, which may benefit the physical and overall experience of cancer and its treatment.

When I received the diagnosis, the colorectal surgeon told me, "I want you to keep all your body parts." I wasn't going to have surgery, only chemotherapy and radiation ("Nigro protocol"). I found myself wanting to know the prognosis. I wanted to know what the chances were of me beating this cancer. I wanted to know the chance of survival. Both the radiation oncologist and medical oncologist said my chances of a cure (both used this word!) were very good—about 70%. Survival rates are based on the number of people who live a minimum of five years after treatment. Some people don't get hung up on the numbers. There are outliers, people who live way beyond the five years. Some people live with stage 4 cancer, the last stage (there is no stage 5), for many years. I know of someone who was treated for anal cancer 18 years ago, and she is doing well. Also, as my oncologist said, there are always advancements in cancer treatments, so if cancer recurs, there will be new ways to tackle it, such as advancements in immunotherapy.

The way society looks at cancer is much like an enemy, a force to be reckoned with. The "War on Cancer" started in the early 1970s and continues to this day. We fight cancer; we want to beat it, and those who fight it are called warriors. This combative approach to cancer is unique, as we don't go to war with multiple sclerosis or acne. It puts us in a victor or loser situation, which can be intimidating in and of itself. I am not the combative type, but I jumped on the "fight" train just like everyone else. In hindsight, I would have much rather preferred to be "treating cancer" and "ridding myself of it," much like someone who wants to remove a tattoo they no longer want.

Financial Issues

Depending on where you live, the medical system may be in your favor or against it. In Canada, most of our treatments (chemoradiation) are covered by our provincial healthcare systems. If we pay for additional coverage, we may also benefit from an extended healthcare plan. Essentials like chemotherapy, radiation therapy, surgery, medications, and hospitalizations may break the bank for someone without health insurance in the United States of America (USA). I have heard of many people in the USA having to not only struggle with their health issues but also battle with the insurance company to see if the costs of expensive treatments will be covered or not.

If you find it too difficult to work, you will need to explore your income options. For me, I had accrued sick leave, plus my employee short-term disability program gave me 67% of my salary. I paid into the program, so it was beneficial to me. You may or may not be fortunate enough to have this program available to you. You may have financial issues to begin with and then decide (or loved ones decide) to start a personal cancer fundraising or online crowdfunding campaign (such as "GoFundMe"). You may also consider organizing a fundraiser to help cover the costs of cancer treatments.

There may be other unexpected costs that come up such as hospital parking costs when you attend appointments, traveling, food, and accommodations if the treatment center or specialists are not near your home. Your family may have to take time off work or be unavailable to work, which can affect their income.

Having the added stress of financial, insurance, or work issues can be alleviated by looking into your options.

Practical Stuff I Wish I Had Known

In hindsight, there were a few things that happened I wished I had known about ahead of time. I was on medical leave for almost nine months.

1. I belong to a professional social work association. I could have put my membership into a "non-practicing" category, and they would have suspended my professional development requirements and reduced my membership fees for the months I was not working.
2. I could have cancelled my parking pass at work and saved myself a couple of hundred dollars.
3. I could have changed my car insurance coverage to indicate I was using it only for pleasure (instead of using it for "all-purpose" to include using my car for work).
4. I could have collected all my medical bills, parking receipts, etc. and claimed them on my insurance/income tax return.

There may be other things I could have done to save myself a few dollars, but unfortunately, I didn't know about them. Think about some of the things you may be able to do to save yourself some money and trouble.

How to Cope

There are many emotions and reactions people experience when they find out they have cancer. If things start to get too upsetting or stressful, you may want to consider counseling or a support group.

Some counselors specialize in cancer-related issues (e.g., social workers, psychologists, psychiatrists).

In one study done in India (Ghoshal, Miriyala, Elangovan, & Rai, 2016), 89 people newly diagnosed with cancer reported the following distressing symptoms (rounded up):

✓ Anxiety (98%)
✓ Depression (90%)
✓ Tiredness (90%)
✓ Pain (87%)
✓ Loss of appetite (70%)

In a study done on the supportive care needs of the person newly diagnosed with cancer (Whelan et. al., 1997), the additional following needs and concerns were found:

✓ Informational needs (85%)
✓ Social concerns (66%)
✓ Need for assistance with day-to-day living (41%)

If you find yourself dealing with any of the previously noted concerns, know you are not alone. It is completely acceptable and normal to react however you do. Coping with and dealing with these stressors and concerns sometimes takes help from others; some you can manage on your own. If you have access to the Internet, you can search for articles and videos regarding any of these strategies that may help you. It's the uncertainty and other stressors that can add up. Each phase of cancer treatment has transitions that can be difficult (more on this in a later chapter).

Here are some examples of ways to help you cope:

- Mindfulness exercises
- Meditation
- Practicing self-affirmations (see Appendix A)
- Writing in a journal
- Prayer or church/synagogue/temple attendance
- Physical activity and exercise
- Getting adequate rest and sleep

Other helpful strategies that may work for you:

- Focus on your well-being
- Be your own advocate and speak up for yourself
- Find positive things in every day (write them down in a journal perhaps?)
- Watch funny movies, TV shows, videos (laughter is good medicine)
- Get outside for some fresh air and sunshine
- Try essential oils in a diffuser (e.g., lavender or citrus)
- Cuddle with a pet (dogs are great for this, and you can even borrow someone else's!)
- Ask for a hug
- Ask for help when you need it
- Seek out expressive arts—paint, draw, dance, play music, etc.
- Realize there will be ups and downs (hopefully the downs won't last too long)
- Take things day by day, hour by hour, moment by moment (baby steps)
- Don't look too far ahead as that can be overwhelming; stay in the present moment
- Assume the treatment is successful
- Get a stuffed animal
- Get a new cozy blanket
- Read inspirational books and stories
- Don't spend too much time alone; for example, if you are bedridden, arrange for someone to be with you during mealtimes

Components of Cancer Grief

You may find yourself feeling very sad, crying, or consumed with thoughts of fear and dread. You may get angry. All these reactions are entirely normal. Grief and loss may overwhelm you. Elizabeth Kübler-Ross has defined five stages of grief, and based on her work, we can understand the emotional pain some people experience with a cancer diagnosis.

Some people with cancer experience components of grief that include the following:

> ➢ Denial (I don't believe it's happening),
> ➢ Anger (Why me? Why now? Anger at the hospital staff, others, self. Anger at the doctor for not diagnosing it sooner),
> ➢ Bargaining (If I am a better person, If I pray more, If I stop eating sugar—I will live through this),
> ➢ Depression (Profound sadness, emptiness, lack of future thinking, suicidal thoughts such as I wish I wouldn't wake up),
> ➢ Acceptance (I have cancer; I will accept whatever happens to me).

Other components of this painful emotional experience could include frustration (at the hospital system, the slow pace of healing and treatment, issues with finances, insurance or work). Fear is also an important component for many. Fear is a strong feeling of the impending loss of something. Fearing for your life or your future can be a terrifying component of cancer grief. Fear can cause crippling anxiety. Grieving anticipated losses can also cause sadness. Grieving for our previous healthy self and "normal" life can be very traumatic.

Feeling shame, guilt, or blaming yourself for thinking you have caused your cancer or ignored the signs can all play parts in your grief experience. Some may feel God is punishing them for doing something or thinking something horrible (or sinful) in the past. Although some of us want to know the cause of our anal cancer, it is not helpful or healthy to believe our cancer was self-inflicted. The stigma and shame associated with this kind of cancer needs to stop. Many people I know do not fit into any of the risk categories for getting anal cancer.

You may also experience survivor's guilt. That's when you know there are others who have experienced cancer, but they don't survive it. We can feel guilty just because we are still alive, and others didn't make it.

Some people's cancer experience can be so difficult (in Body-Mind-Spirit) that it can result in post-traumatic stress disorder (PTSD). Being aware that we don't know how we will react, but hoping for the best is an excellent way to approach the situation.

Not everyone will experience all of these components, and it will not come in the same order for everyone. Your experience will be unique to you. You may go in and out of different stages, and you may have overlapping and mixed emotions at times. One person I know was angry due to the lack of information on anal cancer and has now made it his mission to educate and advocate about the issue. (You can read more about Calvin's story in a later chapter.)

It's important to work through these cancer grief components and try not to repress them. Holding back our feelings can cause added stress. Talk, yell, scream, or cry if you have to. Talking to a counselor or trusted friend, sharing in a support group, or journaling can help you through.

Supports

Some people will decide to keep their cancer diagnosis to themselves. They will turn inward. Sometimes this strategy can cause more stress, difficulties, and poor coping. They may find themselves more isolated. For others, this is the way they cope best after they consider the alternatives. Others will be open about some things and keep other experiences private.

Who do you tell about your cancer? Those who choose to disclose their diagnosis and treatment may find great comfort in that. Family and friends will be well-meaning and will offer to help in any way they can. Often they will feel helpless and worried. If you can let your family and friends know what you need, they will feel like they are helping you. Helping you can make them feel better. It's mutually beneficial.

For instance, early on in my cancer encounter, I asked for my family and friends to tell me stories of people who had overcome cancer and were doing well. I told them I didn't want to hear about people who had died due to a cancer diagnosis. The positive stories were very comforting and gave me hope.

There is a delicate balance between keeping your health status private and sharing your concerns with others to get the support you need. Ask people to keep it to themselves if privacy is important to you.

I told my family and friends that emails and text messages were preferred over phone calls. Phone calls seemed too confrontational or intrusive. If I did talk to someone on the phone, it was at a time that I felt ready for it. Sometimes I broke down in tears, making it difficult to speak. When people sent me messages, it was very kind of them, and it took the pressure off when they said, "No need to respond."

Writing my progress in an online private journal helped me enjoy the real, in-person time with family and friends. Instead of rehashing and going over everything I was experiencing, we were able to focus on nice things, such as watching a funny movie together. I enjoyed them updating me on what was going on in their lives. I appreciated our time together as an opportunity for me not to have to think about my illness.

In addition to in-person support groups, there is a lot of support to be garnered through social media. For example, Facebook has anal cancer groups and cancer support groups. These can be extremely helpful as they provide a community of peers who understand the experience. While enduring the cancer diagnosis, treatment, recovery, and beyond, it's nice to be able to maintain a social life and support network, especially when it's difficult to get out to meet with people face-to-face.

I found a group on Facebook that offered me a lot of support during my anal cancer treatment. I also joined some survivors of cancer groups, which I found to be very helpful. It's nice to be with people (even if it's in a virtual world) who can understand where you are coming from.

You may have people tell you how strong you are and that you are brave. They may see strength in you. You may not feel that. What they see is a person who is undergoing a very stressful, life-threatening experience. It is frightening to them. When there is no other choice, you have to do what you have to do. The will to live is powerful; we go through cancer treatment not only for ourselves but for others.

The most important source of support is yourself. I would encourage you to be self-compassionate, caring, and loving toward yourself—the same as you would be to a best friend. Foster self-love and patience with yourself. Set aside time for expressing and honoring all your feelings, and give yourself time to go through the process. Let your feelings just BE. Acknowledge and accept them. As much as you want it all to be over, your body (and mind) needs time to heal.

Give yourself a break from worrying about the house, car, or kids looking perfect. Don't worry about the clutter, the housekeeping, or the laundry. Let someone else worry about these things for you. Things may end up being done differently, but that's okay, as long as they are getting done.

Consider finding someone else to shop or cook for you if those tasks are challenging. Maybe you need someone to look after the kids while you are at appointments. Call on your friends for these kinds of things. They will enjoy feeling needed.

You may be lucky enough to find a peer, mentor, or "Cancer Buddy." A peer is someone who has gone through a similar experience and wants to help answer your questions, coach, support, and encourage you through your cancer ordeal. The peer support person is in a better position to understand you and help you cope. Your Cancer Buddy may also have some great answers to your questions or be able to guide you to the right person to get the answers.

Words of Caution—Protect yourself from those who mean well by forwarding all kinds of alternative or natural cures your way. There will be some people who will not respect your decision to have conventional treatments (chemo and radiation, for example) and vice versa. You will also want to protect yourself from people who are nosy versus genuinely caring and kind people who wish nothing but the best for your well-being.

Notes From a Cancer Support Buddy

Cindy Ring

When I was going through this horrible ordeal, I was blindsided. I felt alone and had no one to compare experiences with. No one could relate to what I was going through. My dad would ask me how I was feeling. When I was honest, his facial expressions of how hurt he felt broke my heart. Afterwards, I just told him I felt great.

At work, only a few friends and supervisors knew I was sick. I had an extraordinary support system of family members taking my child to school in the morning while my brother took me to my radiation appointments. Friends took me to medical appointments for reconstruction surgery due to the aftermath of the radiation. But all this time I felt alone, as no one could relate.

I decided to become a peer support to others with anal cancer because I wanted to help by giving them insight regarding what was to come and to be there for them when needed, even if it was just to talk or have someone to cry with. I can relate to what someone else is going through to help them win their fight against cancer. Having a solid support system helps motivate anyone to fight hard.

The difficulty with being a cancer support buddy is that you are unable to be there physically for your buddy through this heartache. Your buddies are usually in different states or countries.

Not knowing what was happening to me with the extensive side effects and what was to come after the completion of treatment was absolutely the worst thing I had ever experienced. Being there for someone else going through the same or similar ordeal makes me feel happy that they are not alone. They will always know they have someone who cares.

Sharing Updates of Tests, Treatments and Well-Being

Depending on whom you tell about your cancer diagnosis, there may be few or many people who want to stay updated on your progress and condition. If you happen to be blessed with many caring individuals in your life, you may have a group of people who are concerned about your well-being. The phone could be ringing a lot, or you may have to answer a lot of messages on the computer or your phone.

There are ways to get around the stress of needing to tell many people the same thing. You can assign a point person, or someone who can take those calls for you. You can put your updates on social media, such as Facebook. For those who want more privacy, you can make a private Facebook page so only those invited to the group will see the posts. The problem with this is that not everyone is on Facebook.

What I ended up doing was making a private online blog. Only those who had been invited to see my online journal were able to access it. An email went out when I posted an update. Sometimes it was daily. Sometimes my daughter had to write the post for me because I was not well enough. This process worked very well for me. When I felt comfortable, and I knew I was ready to share it more widely, I posted parts of my story on social media. I received a lot of support, and it helped immensely.

Passing the Time

There will be some points in your cancer experience where you will be waiting. Waiting for tests, waiting for results, and waiting for the treatment to get started can be anxiety-provoking. It seems to me the most difficult time, psychologically, is between diagnosis and waiting for treatment to begin. While we are waiting, there are many things we can do to pass the time, especially if we are not able to work or keep active. Sometimes it helps to have a purpose or things to distract you.

Here are some ideas that can help pass the time and keep your mind on other things:

- Adult coloring books
- Writing
- Drawing
- Listening to or playing music
- Watching TV, movies
- Sleeping
- Reading—especially light-hearted or "easy read" books and magazines
- Puzzle books—crossword, word search, Sudoku
- Deck of cards—solitaire or play games with family or friends
- Games on a handheld device such as a phone or tablet

(More on how I coped in a later chapter.)

Assembling Your Healthcare/Oncology Team (a.k.a. Your Team)

Doctors, specialists, nurses, allied health professionals, family members, and friends will form "your team." This cancer journey cannot be taken alone. When you find out who is there for your needs and what role they have, make sure you write it down. Ask for a business card and jot down a note or two on it. There may be an after-hours number you can call if something comes up in the evenings or weekends, and there may be an urgent cancer care clinic you can visit. Determining who to call and for what purpose takes a bit of time to figure out.

On my team I had a colorectal surgeon, radiation oncologist, medical oncologist, radiation nurse, oncology nurse, family doctor, a nurse at the family doctor's office, gynecologist, social worker, dietician, priest, psychologist/friend, psychiatrist, husband, son, daughter, mom, dad, close friends, and extended family members. I also had many friends from work, acquaintances, family friends, Facebook friends, etc. This all helped me cope with my upcoming cancer ordeal.

Your team will comprise some of those listed above, as well as others I didn't have. These people will be there for you, and knowing whom to call on and for what reason is key to feeling supported and cared for.

Another helpful tip is to make sure you write down your non-urgent questions for the team so when you attend appointments, you won't forget to ask. Audio recording your visits or bringing someone along with you can also be helpful, as often we miss things. Make sure to ask about medication refills or prescriptions, follow-ups, and next steps. (More on keeping organized a bit later.)

Preparing for Treatment

If you work, you may want to arrange for some time off to go through your treatments. For me, I had already been on sick leave due to some complications I was experiencing. I've known others who were able to work throughout their treatment, so it may take a wait-and-see approach.

You may want to take a break from some of your obligations and responsibilities. For example, you can put volunteer commitments you have on hold. Reduce the extra stress of other little jobs by delegating someone else to look after things for a while.

Knowledge is power. Read through any literature you receive on kitchen and food safety, nutrition, coping with cancer, information on chemotherapy and radiation therapy, or any other booklets or articles you are given. You may want to share some of these with your family members.

You may want to do everything you can to clear your schedule so you can look after you. If you have young children or sick or older parents, you may find this hard, but with some creative thinking and organizing, it can be managed. The focus is now on you. For some of us, this is a very foreign concept, as we are used to taking care of other people. Now is the time for us to be taken care of.

If there are toxic or stressful people in your life, you will want to avoid them over the next few months. The less stress in your life, the better.

Once the treatment plan is in motion, there is a need for preparation. A CT simulation (a test-run) may be required. I was asked to have a full bladder for this appointment (feeling like I needed to go to the toilet, but not uncomfortable). The full bladder is essential because it helps with target localization and reduces the risk of injury to the bladder and the small bowel by pushing them away from the radiation field. Once the radiation team positioned me as I lay under the scanner on my back, they tattooed a small black dot onto each hip. Some people get it done with a black marker, which they don't wash off until the end of treatment. The marking helped ensure I was in the correct position for each radiation treatment. The clerk gave me my appointment schedule for radiation and chemotherapy on a week-to-week basis.

I went to the hospital to have a peripherally inserted central catheter (PICC) put into my right upper arm. A long tube was inserted into my vein. This allowed easy access to my blood for testing, and it also provided quick and painless administration of chemotherapy or other medications. It reduced the necessity for needle pokes. Alternatively, you may get a port in your upper chest. I wore a pump, or "baby bottle," around my neck for 96 hours as the medicine was slowly infused into my body.

I was told to keep myself well and strong and to make sure I was eating a healthy diet. I had a meeting with the dietician, and my family also attended so they could help make sure I was getting the nutrition I needed moving forward.

I had meetings with the medical oncologist and the pharmacist regarding side effects of chemotherapy and what to watch for concerning the medication I would receive. There may be some antinausea medications (to help prevent nausea or a sick feeling) you can start even before your treatment begins. It's important to let the doctor and pharmacist know everything you are taking, including vitamins, herbs, and supplements. Some of these products can interfere with chemotherapy or other cancer treatments and the healing process. Don't assume because it's natural it's safe.

I met with the radiation therapist to go over what to watch for regarding side effects. They explained what I should expect and told me they were there for me if any issues or questions came up.

Starting Treatment

Your treatment may include chemotherapy, radiation therapy, surgery, or a combination of these. You may want someone with you when you attend your first chemotherapy and radiation therapy appointments. Sticking to your schedule will give you the best chance of eliminating cancer.

Your team will be monitoring your progress. Your blood will be taken. They will ask you how you are doing. Be as honest as you can about your pain levels, symptoms, mood, energy and sleep patterns, appetite, and ability to cope. If you have any complications, you may be hospitalized for more intensive treatment. Sometimes people are given a break for a while so their body can heal a bit and get stronger before resuming treatments.

Untoward Treatment Side Effects

As I mentioned previously, everyone's cancer is different. Every body is unique. Therefore, everyone's reaction to treatment will vary (see the chapter on Anal Cancer Basics for more information on side effects). Some will have little to no side effects, others will have moderate effects. Those who are unfortunate will endure great suffering.

I was one of the unfortunate ones. I ended up in the hospital due to "febrile neutropenia" (a fever plus low white blood cells). The chemotherapy brought my white blood cell count down, and I developed an infection. I had to be hospitalized, and I received antibiotics intravenously. Spending over a week in the hospital, I received many antibiotics as well as a blood transfusion. Frequently, if blood counts are low, a transfusion of platelets or red blood cells can help one feel much better. It's not complicated; the blood transfusion is administered through the vein attached to the PICC line or port. This happens to many people who go through chemoradiation, and the doctors and other health professionals always stay on top of this, watching for signs of adverse effects.

Sexuality for both men and women may change. Most people who go through any cancer treatment experience changes in that area. For those undergoing anal cancer treatment, radiation targets the sensitive pelvic region, and there could be resulting physical sexual problems that need to be addressed. There could also be changes in hormones for women. Mentally and emotionally, there could be a change in sexual feelings toward a partner, and there may be a lack of interest in sexual relations as treatment and recovery proceeds. If you are having concerns in any of these areas, it's important to have a discussion with your healthcare provider to ensure your concerns are adequately addressed.

A note about fecal incontinence (poop accidents): Dr. Foster Lasley, a radiation oncologist, states he has noticed if people develop fecal incontinence before starting radiation it probably won't get better. If the accidents develop during or shortly after radiation, then sometimes it can get better as people heal from radiation side effects. He said Kegel exercises (squeezing your anal muscles) might help a little—usually not a lot though. I would also like to add that a pelvic floor physiotherapist may be able to offer some help with fecal incontinence.

Moving Forward Toward Treatment and Recovery

Once you feel well-armed and prepared to deal with your cancer diagnosis and treatment, things might come up that you weren't expecting. It's always important to keep in mind that "unexpected things" can happen. The day after my first chemoradiation treatment, I phoned the urgent cancer clinic and spoke to a nurse. I told her my heart was racing. I asked her if this was "normal." She replied by saying, "When dealing with cancer and its treatment, nothing is normal." She reassured me by saying that unless I was feeling faint, light-headed, or having chest pain, I should be all right. And I was.

I took advantage of all programs offered through our local cancer care facility. The library had a great selection of books. I especially enjoyed the free "Look Good Feel Better" program for women and enjoyed all the makeup, lotions and other goodies I came home with!

Keeping Organized

It's important to keep all your appointments, reports, information sheets and booklets, instructions, phone numbers, etc. in an easy-to-locate spot. Some store phone numbers and business cards in a phone book. Others put them into their cell phones. A binder, bag or folder keeps things together and is easy to access when needed.

On the website of the hospital I was attending, I found out about a booklet called "My Cancer Notebook." It is a small spiral-bound notebook with space to record health information, doctor's phone numbers, appointments, etc. It is a great way to keep things organized. I have also seen other cancer treatment planners, so there may be one that works for you.

When I was going through treatment and in the early days of recovery, I had many things to remember to do. There was medication to take, nutritional supplements, baking soda baths four times daily, creams, radiation therapy appointments, chemotherapy appointments, specialist appointments, etc. My daughter, Simone, helped me with this by designing an appointment/care schedule on a whiteboard. All I had to do was refer to the board for things I needed to do, then place a check mark in the required box when done. This helped keep me on track.

Reminders on my cell phone and sharing my appointment dates and times with others helped me secure rides and companionship/support to appointments.

Preparing for my second week of chemotherapy, I cleared my schedule of any unnecessary activities and rescheduled appointments (with my gynecologist and dentist, for example).

Things You May Need

There were things I needed to have close at hand. I had some of this stuff already, and some I needed to purchase or borrow. I found out about what I may need by talking to others about how they dealt with some of the same kinds of side effects.

Here is a list of supplies you may want to consider for your safety, comfort, and healthcare management (see Appendix B for a more comprehensive list):

- Digital thermometer
- Memory foam® topper for mattress
- Washable soaker pads
- Washable cotton pads (I made mine out of flannel baby blankets)
- Depend® disposable briefs, sanitary napkins
- Mesh pants
- Sensitive skin baby wipes
- Barrier creams and wipes
- Moisturizing lotion
- Hand sanitizer
- Lip balm
- Biotene® mouthwash
- Healing ointments (e.g., Aquaphor®)
- Nutritional supplement drinks (e.g., Boost®/Ensure®)
- Latex gloves
- Finger cots (latex cover for the fingertip)
- Baking soda
- Plastic home sitz bath

Medications you may want to inquire about:

- "Magic mouthwash" (to treat or prevent mouth sores or thrush)
- Analgesics (for pain)
- Antinausea medications
- Sleeping pills
- Antidepressants
- Creams to help with radiation burns (e.g., Silvadene®/ Flamazine®)

If there are any difficulties or concerns you run up against, don't delay talking to your medical team. They will have some suggestions or advice for you. They will also know what can counteract your treatment, so it is important to discuss these treatments ahead of time. For example, the nurse instructed me to ensure all creams, lotions, and medications were cleaned off my bottom area before radiation therapy because if I didn't, they could cause increased burns. Also, some say to not put anything on your bottom area for at least 1-2 hours after radiation treatment (think of it as a sunburn; the burning continues even when you get out of the sun). Another tip I received was to put ice chips in my mouth during the chemotherapy push to help avoid mouth sores. It worked!

Positive Side of Cancer

I know it is hard to think of cancer from a positive viewpoint, but in time I hope you will gain some incredible insight regarding your life. For me, I learned about who really cared about me and how much I was loved and appreciated. I learned about the importance of genuine love and compassion for those who are suffering or grieving. I learned how strong I am and how the will to live is greater than I knew. I learned about the fragility of life and how important it is to enjoy every moment of every day as much as possible.

In the face of my mortality, I learned how to prioritize my life and transform myself. I became much closer to God. I look at life and death very differently now and appreciate every moment I am alive on this earth. Some people say it's a blessing to have cancer, while others say everything happens for a reason. For me, this was a random event, and I dug hard to see what I could learn from it. I have come out an enriched, spiritual, awakened soul.

Helping Others Can Help You

For the most part, it is very difficult to help others when a person is dealing with cancer and treatment. However, if you ever find yourself in a position where you can offer a sympathetic or compassionate ear to someone facing a similar experience, it may be helpful. Mutual support is key to our human connections and feeling good about others and ourselves. When we can share our insights, blessings, and lessons with others, it can offer the inspiration others may need to find hope, joy, and love in their everyday. Others may end up sharing with you how your diagnosis has made them reflect on their mortality and how much they appreciate and love you. Sharing these mutual feelings can deepen your relationships moving forward. You will have a new appreciation for how you can help others through troubling or stressful times.

Being Prepared Can Help You Cope

If we are prepared for the worst and hope for the best, we have a better chance of successfully coping with and dealing with cancer and its treatment. I am assuming because you are reading this chapter that like me, you want to be prepared. Cancer affects us holistically—Body-Mind-Spirit. Knowing the good, the bad, and the ugly can help settle our anxieties about the uncertainty.

****

REFERENCES:

Ghoshal, S., Miriyala, R., Elangovan, A., & Rai, B. (2016). Why Newly Diagnosed Cancer Patients Require Supportive Care. An Audit from a Regional Care Center in India. *Indian Journal of Palliative Care*, 22(3), 326-330.

Kübler-Ross, E., & Kessler, D. (2005). *On Grief and Grieving: Finding the meaning of grief through the five stages of loss.* New York: Toronto: Scribner.

Whelan, T. J., Mohide, E. A, Willan, A. R., Arnold, A., Tew, M., Sellick, S., Gafni, A., & Levine, M. N. (1997). The Supportive Care Needs of Newly Diagnosed Cancer Patients Attending a Regional Care Center. *Cancer*, 80(8). https://doi.org/10.1002/(SICI)1097-0142(19971015)80:8<1518::AID-NCR21>3.0.CO;2-7.

Chapter 3

No One Should Suffer Alone

A sister's perspective by Crystal

Sometime around 1980, my mother told me my older sister, Ashley, had cancer. She didn't tell me what type of cancer or where the cancer was. I was in school and had the flexibility to stay with my sister to support and keep her company. She refused my offer, and I was confused. So although I lived a distance away, I took several buses to visit her multiple times a week. My visits needed to be short (she wouldn't let me stay longer than about an hour). A nurse came to see her daily, and I had to leave before the nurse arrived.

It was months later when Ashley told me she had a form of anal cancer. She didn't go into detail, and I didn't want to pry—she was clearly uncomfortable talking about it. I tried to make sense of it on my own. It took me a while to figure out what was going on for her (in the days before Google) and what she must be enduring—especially after radical surgery. Ashley did not speak to me about it, and as far as I know, she didn't speak to anyone else either. I eventually learned she had a colostomy, and she spoke to me a few times about it being a hassle to manage (meaning to keep it clean).

Many years later we started walking together regularly. She could keep up a good pace and was considered fully recovered. She did not speak of the cancer, the surgery, or her "bag." Walking together is one of those activities that tended to invite confidences. It was many years later Ashley told me of the suffering she had endured after the surgery and continued to endure because the site of the wound had never fully healed.

Ashley told me her doctor made a horrible comment to her when she was diagnosed, which chilled any urge she had to share and filled her with shame. She did not tell me exactly what he said, but she shared that he didn't seem to be focused on the right things, which also delayed her diagnosis. She said he seemed to be more interested in trying to figure out how and why she had the cancer in the first place.

Ashley is 15 years older than me. I was an adult when this happened to her. I think of how differently she coped when compared to my mother, who'd had breast cancer. My mother was very sociable, and all of us were involved in her care back then. Mother was spiritual and read and breathed books about the healing power of love. She drank water out of a red glass that had sat in the sun for 24 hours.

My sister and I are no longer close, and as I write this, I think of her quietly, stoically suffering alone. Maybe even today she quietly endures. She has survived this cancer. Writing this has given me occasion to wonder if her suffering would have been less if she had been able to share it. I can't help but wonder what it could have been like for her without the stigma and shame associated with anal cancer.

Chapter 4

Stuff No One Told Me!

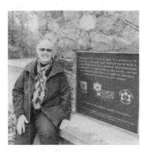

Sharon Basic

I believe there are many different kinds of reactions to being told one has cancer. I dealt with the diagnosis in a matter-of-fact way. Immediately after waking up from the colonoscopy, I was told I had cancer, not a hemorrhoid, and because of its location, I might need surgery, a colostomy, and cancer treatment. I would be referred to the cancer center and a colorectal surgeon. My response was, "Oh, my husband had a colostomy. I can deal with that!"

It's not that the word "cancer" did not frighten me. I had peace of mind that what will be will be. Let me explain. I am older, not mature—just older. I was 67 at the time, and I had seen and been through a lot. The word cancer was not new to me.

My mother died of cancer in 1978. I was a caregiver to my husband for seven years as he bravely dealt with colorectal cancer and died in 2006. He had three major surgeries before the cancer metastasized to his brain. So I knew a lot about colostomies, chemo, and radiation cancer treatments. That kind of knowledge is terribly insufficient compared to actually going through it. In my opinion, being a caregiver is far more emotionally difficult than being a patient!

My husband and I cried for each other. I cried for him and myself because of my fear of losing him and being alone. He cried for me, not wanting to leave me alone. He was incredibly strong and accepted his fate.

After the MRI and the biopsy report, there was utter relief I did not have colorectal cancer. I had squamous cell anal cancer and was told the treatment was highly successful, and the recurrence rate was very low. Often no surgery was required. However, the disease had traveled to one lymph node in the groin, and there was one other questionable lymph node. There is one tiny spot on the lung they are still watching, but it is considered to be scar tissue from pneumonia I had as a youngster.

Having cancer sometimes means you have to deal with comforting others. In fact, I had to comfort my friend who received the news along with me immediately on waking up from the colonoscopy. She drove me home and then broke into tears—I hugged her and told her it would be all right!

Treatment

Treatment is not pleasant by any means, but I told myself thousands have been through it before me and were survivors—I can be a survivor too!

Chemotherapy made me very sick! The only diet I could manage was rice and chicken. To this day I cannot cook chicken. The smell turns my stomach. I lost 35 pounds over the course of treatment. I required a weekly infusion of fluids. This I blame on not receiving antinausea medication soon enough. Looking back, I should have been prescribed them and started taking them even before I started treatment. I had severe diarrhea and relied heavily on medication. Near the end, I wore Depends® when going out to appointments. I still keep a supply of Depends® in my emergency kit in my car. I always took towels with me. I sat on towels. I slept on towels.

I had wonderful, supportive friends and family through treatment and recovery. I was especially fortunate to have two nieces with me for the appointments with the surgeon, medical oncologist (chemotherapy), and radiation doctor appointments. One of my nieces, Leesa, is a veterinarian, and the other, Rhonda, is a nurse, so their knowledge and support were invaluable (even though as my Power of Attorney for medical care, I tease that between the two, I could easily be put down for a hangnail!) It was important to know what questions to ask. It was also helpful to have someone who was well-informed attend the appointments with me.

I'd like to share one of my favorite radiation stories that we still hysterically laugh about today. One day I was waiting for my radiation treatment with one of the girls. I was sipping on my water, desperately trying to get enough down. I turned a bit green and said I felt sick. My niece asked me if I needed the wastebasket, and I said "No." No sooner had I gotten that out when I rushed to the wastebasket, threw up, and peed myself! A couple of ladies from the hospital were passing by, and they rushed to get me towels to clean up and made a big fuss. They helped me back to my seat, beside my niece—who sat there almost laughing! I sent her out to the car to get my change of clothes I always had with me. After that, I always carried the backpack with me. Duh . . . what good was it out in the car? Lesson learned. I got changed and had my treatment (obviously without the required full bladder). We laughed and laughed about it on the way home. It did teach me to carry the change of clothes with me (and there are still clothes in the car to this day!).

My nieces and my friends helped a lot at my home when I was too weak to do my chores. At times they had to help with messy laundry and followed behind me cleaning up! I appreciated the help with yard work, housework, and fixing meals for the freezer. Leesa stayed with me overnight the last few days of treatment. She then went back to Stratford in the morning to go to work. The last night home she woke me up every two hours to check my temperature. She called Rhonda and said I had to be taken to the Cancer Center in the morning. I was very weak, burned from the radiation, and had to be put into a wheelchair. I was admitted to the hospital (more on that later).

To this day, Rhonda continues to fill my freezer with healthy meals! I have a fragile digestive system, and she knows what kinds of food I can tolerate.

What No One Told Me!

I talked to a teacher friend, an anal cancer survivor herself, about the upcoming treatment I would receive. She told me she informed her principal she would come back to work when she could wear underwear again! Wow, did I laugh at that, only to find out that commando style and skirts were my best friends.

Radiation can cause a lot of burned skin in the pelvic area. Those 25 radiation treatments severely burned me. Underwear was out of the question! Modesty made me hesitant to complain loudly enough until it was so bad I refused any more treatment. I was unfortunate enough to be so badly burned that I spent 14 days in the hospital for treatment (not the three to five days they predicted). Chemotherapy was completed, but I missed the last five radiation treatments. Treatment ended on July 20, 2015.

It was a long time before I could comfortably wear underwear or tight pants again. Luckily it was summertime, so I did not have to deal with cold breezes!

Another thing no one told me is radiation causes total hair loss, but not on my head, mind you. I experienced pubic hair loss, which has been semi-permanent. That meant some complications with urinating—more of a spray than a stream! Extra toilet seat cleaning is needed. The hair on my head did become thinner, I believe from the lack of nutrition, nausea, and diarrhea I experienced.

I was informed about the side effects of radiation on the bowels. However, it took two years before I found a relatively reliable solution to my bowel incontinence. A couple of sessions with a dietician, which I should have insisted on earlier, gave me the information I needed to cope. On telling the chemo doctor about my dietary success, I was told I was lucky, as a lot of patients don't ever recuperate after bowel radiation. For me, the simple solution was having oatmeal every morning!

Nerve pains were shooting down my leg for at least a year. My family doctor told me young people heal faster . . . LOL . . . but not to worry!

At times I was so weak I had to use a walker. I couldn't do any stairs, and walking a few steps every day was a challenge. In fact, when I went outside, I did use the walker and stubbornly each day did a bit more. My goal was to be able to walk far enough to be able to go out to one of my favorite home furnishing stores. In fact, it was the first store a friend took me to. I used a cart for support, and it was enough for that trip out. It was quite a while before I could attempt a larger warehouse store.

Through my Retired Teachers Insurance Plan, there is a program called "The CAREpath Navigation System, Survivor Support Program and Cancer Information Line." I was assigned an oncology nurse and talked to her weekly on the phone. She had access to my medical records, the test results, and doctors' reports. She could translate and advise me. She gave me ideas on how to deal with the side effects. I still talk to her after every doctor's appointment— which are three months apart now. Now I see either the radiation or chemotherapy doctor or surgeon every three months.

Moving Forward

The radiologist told me the chance the anal cancer would return was less than 1%. However, the follow-up CT scans and scopes are always stressful. The radiation doctor does a thorough check of my lymph nodes, neck, and groin. He also checks my lungs and liver. And, of course, the finger-check of the anus. There is one rough spot that was questionable in the beginning, after treatment, but it has smoothed out and is considered to be nothing to worry about. The surgeon said there was nothing to biopsy. The chemo doctor does a similar check. Depending on the specialist, I am seen every 3-6 months.

I had an external hemorrhoid pop up, and I was referred to the surgeon earlier than the regular three-month check, just in case. At every visit, she does an anoscopy of the anal area. It isn't considered a full scope. It is minimally invasive, and no bowel cleaning preparation is needed. I like to watch on the monitor, and I learn a lot as she describes what she sees to the resident (I attend a teaching hospital). She has a very matter-of-fact way about her. She said (perhaps for the resident's sake as well as mine), "We are going to have a look. It may be the cancer returning, it may be new cancer, or it may be a hemorrhoid." Some may not like her frank manner, but I respect, like, and trust her so much. She confirmed the exterior lump is a hemorrhoid. I know when it developed. I had a rough day after eating too much mango and was on the toilet many times that day. By the way, the treatment she gave me was to have two warm baths a day—thank you!

I had an optional CT scan of my chest and abdomen two years after treatment. All was okay, at least no changes.

I am almost two and a half years from the end of treatment. I appreciate being monitored carefully, but it is a reminder, and I wonder if this checkup will be all clear or not. Are they worried about me? Should I be worried about me? Do they think it will come back? Has it come back? I am on pins and needles until I get the results. My family doctor often calls me immediately to tell me, "All is well."

One remedy for my lowered energy level has been the Vitamin B12 shots my family doctor has prescribed. Was my Vitamin B12 deficiency a result of decreased nutrition, the harsh treatment, or plain old age? I'm not sure, but I do feel better now.

There are so many reminders that keep "cancer thoughts" alive. Driving by the Cancer Center, my mouth would get dry remembering having to force myself to drink the water before my radiation treatment. There were days I would gag on water.

Cancer remains a big part of my life—not like a bout of the flu, my gallbladder surgery, or even my hysterectomy. It is in my choices of what I can and can't do. What I can eat, where I can go, and how I plan my day as I am still fearful of being too far from a washroom. Unfortunately for those around me, it is still in my conversations. Often in a joking manner, but it is there. I try to keep it out of my head and not to voice it as I am sure people don't want to hear it. But it is always lurking there. Sometimes I use it as a crutch and an excuse to explain my behavior or situation. I have had a change in outlook and activity, and I blame it on cancer and treatment. But could it just be laziness? Or just a different attitude on life? If I don't feel like doing something, I don't do it. That part I like!

I didn't realize how some of my relationships with friends and family would change. With some, I have become so much closer, and some relationships have become more strained and distant. We naturally have people come and go throughout our lives. I think cancer magnifies that. We change, and relationships change. I try to keep cancer talk out of conversations, but my change in attitude about life is obvious. Things I liked to do before may not be what is important now. I have become selfish about my time. And I think that is a positive, good thing!

I do have a zest for life! I am a survivor each and every day I am alive. Life is meant to be lived and enjoyed every day. If I desire an afternoon nap, I have an afternoon nap. If I plan to have lunch and go shopping with a friend, that is my priority for the day. Regardless of what we are going through, what fate has in store for us, we have today. Enjoy it!

My advice to those who are going through a similar experience is to surround yourselves with positive friends and family. Think positive thoughts and be grateful for every day!

I am thankful every day, every month, every year that I am a survivor.

I am strong . . . I am a survivor.

Chapter 5

The Shame of Anal Cancer

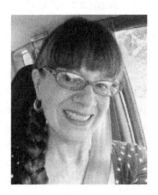

Joana Dougherty McGee

Editor's Note: Based on the original post in "Anal Cancer" closed Facebook group, December 30, 2017.

Does anybody else suffer from the discomfort of addressing the term "anal cancer?" I am saddled with deep complexes that few share to the same degree, which limits me.

I am a very active Facebook (FB) person (as I am sitting in my chair so much of the time!). As a counselor who now works online with people for free, I get many referrals and have many, many people in my everyday FB network. I am rather closed about personal things and never address this cancer because of hang-ups I have never been able to shed.

Strict Roman Catholic Upbringing

Growing up in an absurdly strict and suffocating Roman Catholic family, school, and community, I was taught the body is an "instrument of sin," and everything related to it is vulgar, shameworthy, and disgusting. I will never forget when, in third grade, a boy in the row next to me passed gas. The nun struck him so hard, he fell from his seat. "You disgusting animal!" she bellowed at him.

I had a close friend in the seminary who was molested. Nothing about the body was pure and innocent . . . that is what I learned, and I learned it well. Everything about the body, and ESPECIALLY "down there" was shown to us to be repugnant, vulgar, and profoundly shameful.

I am no longer Catholic, nor exclusively Christian, not by a long shot. And that's okay. I am not in the least concerned that "God" doesn't love me and have no concerns in any spiritual way at ALL. I don't believe such human construct baloney regarding God having conditions about anything in the expression of love.

How I Get Around Using the Word Anal

I have lived my life with these beliefs, and indeed, they have imposed deep limitations on me and on my freedom to be happy in my everyday life.

I firmly believe I aided in my body's development of both bladder and anal (can hardly write it) cancer BECAUSE I held so much shame there. Some might laugh, but I feel it to be absolutely so.

Due to the shame I have always felt about the body, I have found it impossible to ever say that I have had anal cancer. It is too descriptive for me to bear. I mean, "colon cancer," sure. On hearing that, one thinks about the general abdominal area. But "anal cancer," well, one cannot help but think of more graphic pictures. Heck, I cannot even talk about boobs or other things without imploding in embarrassment and discomfort.

50

With professionals, I ALWAYS say exactly what is happening with me physically, using correct terms. I don't play games when it concerns such vital issues; hell, why go at all if you aren't going to be straight with them? So that area's okay.

I am hung up about using the language of this cancer personally, in my life. If I refer to it, I always say that I have had colorectal cancer. It's diffuse and easy. I'm not saying it's the thing to do, just saying it is what I do. I am not ready to break that custom, and that's okay too. Naturally, my family and those closest to me know the score, but that is the extent of it. They know everything.

I am so immature about this, but it is what it is. Interestingly, I work in the health field (with cancer patients!), and I am continually dealing with people whose bodies are doing myriad unsavory things as they struggle forward. Even so, I cannot bear to pronounce the words that properly describe my cancerous past.

I refer to this a LOT, as I work with pediatric cancer patients, and it's always nice for them to know that I get it. If there were a circumstance in which I felt my specifically mentioning anal cancer was important, I would not hesitate. Again, I don't play games if it stands to benefit another significantly. But I won't just offer.

Living With the Fear of Shameful Accidents

Due to surgeon error, I was left with a big gap in my anus–it was entirely unnecessary. I manage it by eating once a day (something I had ALWAYS done, so it was natural . . . and yes, I know it's not very good), "emptying out" in the morning, and then facing my day, always using pads, etc. If I have an accident, it will literally "pour out." No controlling it, as it is coming through a gap.

With 40 radiation treatments and pre-existing gastrointestinal (GI) problems (stage 3 bladder cancer, interstitial cystitis, and colitis), it was assumed I would have extensive problems. I will have the runs for the rest of my life. It is what it is, and that's how I deal with it. My lovely doctor reminds me that whenever I want, I can have a colostomy, but I resist and will continue to resist unless something happens to change this routine for the worst.

51

SO, the main thing is the silly shame with the body words, which I am not ready to get over, and the HORRIBLE shame with friends or family in the event of having an accident. Regarding THAT, I die a thousand times just writing about it here.

There ARE times, however, when I have felt death would have been preferable (than having an accident while with a friend, for example, or while I am at the grocery store cashier). I can barely stand to recall them, and they are horrible nightmares to me.

I envy those who know this is yet another affliction and nothing to be ashamed about. Naturally, it is the correct and mature position.

A Response from Penny—How She Got Over the Shame

"I, also, was raised a devout Catholic, so I can totally relate. I still leave words relating to sex and certain body parts out of sentences when speaking. Here is why I am a little better with it in such a short time.

1. People who care about me aren't going to judge me, and if they do, it isn't about me, it's about them and their insecurities, limitations, and needs.

2. Unlike many others, possibly including you, I probably did cause my cancer by sleeping unprotected with someone in my twenties. Here's the thing: I cannot change my mistake (we all make them). All I can do is try to do better, which I am. I have teenagers. I am trying to teach them to do better than I did.

3. The word anal refers to a body part just like the word breast. Would you feel the same shame if it were breast cancer? Try to become more mechanical with your words, the same way your doctor would. Take the power YOU have given away from that word.

4. I have read and been told by a researcher that HPV is not the only cause of anal cancer. Should someone who got it from benign anal lesions be ashamed also?

5. I, for one, believe that the toughest/most uncomfortable situations are where we find purpose and meaning. I don't know you, but I would be willing to bet you have quite a purpose here. In other words, if your diagnosis and friendship helped to start this group, then thank you. I don't know where I would be without it! (On a side note, I am a recovering Catholic, but still a practicing Christian.) I was just like you. I think we were taught wrong; we are not going to hell because we have anal cancer. That's just silly. God loves us."

Joana's Response to Penny

The mechanical thing is what I need to practice. If it were breast, (I think) it would be fine, particularly in our breast cancer-crazed society. Who knows?

And—you're right about purpose: I have several about which I am deeply passionate. I would hazard a guess that my life purpose and overall philosophy became enriched and grew in beautiful ways when faced with these serious illnesses. It seems through the most difficult situations there is much to be gained; it's almost always been that way for me.

Regarding the Catholicism, it's interesting. My experience was bad, obviously. When all of a sudden, as if dropped from the sky, I was offered a teaching job at a Roman Catholic high school in Berkeley, California, I knew there was a reason this had come to be. Though I wanted to run fast in the other direction, I truly believed I had to take it. I needed to experience something that was being handed to me.

As a Spanish speaker who has worked extensively with refugees from South and Central America, I was also impressed with the priests and nuns there who espoused and acted in association with Liberation Theology. They categorically rejected the filthy rich corruption of the church and responded with pastoral work with the people, guiding them toward lives of dignity (helping build wells or homes, for example). Fabulous work was being done, and I knew several of these priests and nuns back in those days. It was the most WONDERFUL place; people were truly walking the beautiful talk. What a wonderful experience.

Joana's Ability to See the Humor in it All

One funny thing I laugh about with my husband is the rotten "karma" I was dealt! Heck, now when I see a person in a white coat, I automatically either bend over or spread my legs! Tee-hee.

I will never forget when I had a pre-surgery appointment for the bladder cancer. I was so frightened and so embarrassed that I took more tranquilizer than I was accustomed to (I don't take them at all). Totally loopy, I can be very weird (runs in the family!). The drop-dead handsome young doctor came in, and, smiling beautifully down on me, he said, "How are you feeling now? Are you doing okay?" I answered (my husband told me this; I don't even remember), "I am so okay, you could put an elephant's trunk up there and I would be fine!"

All joking aside, the shame remains. Not the young shame of feeling like a horrible sinner—I don't feel that at all. It's simply residual shame that developed into its own thing over a lifetime. I am not terribly concerned with it, as it doesn't rear its head frequently in my everyday life.

Chapter 6

Mental Health, Coping, and Anal Cancer

Angela G. Gentile

Standing at the beginning of the long hallway, looking for the sign that says X-ray Department, you see it—"Mental Health," with an arrow pointing to the right. You think to yourself, "I am glad that's not where I am headed. Those people are crazy."

The concept of "mental health" is one that is still often stigmatized. The word mental can cause some people to imagine a "crazy" person with dirty, messy hair, loud outbursts and unpredictable, anti-social behavior. As a mental health professional, I have come to understand the importance of de-stigmatizing the concepts of impaired psychological, emotional, and cognitive functioning. Mental health problems are usually invisible, and no one is immune to them.

My profession as a clinical social worker has given me the honor and privilege of working with many people who are affected by various forms of mental illness. I have worked primarily with adults, including the older adult population. In the older adult population (those 65 and older), many people are depressed, anxious, and grieving, as well as living with cognitive (thinking and memory) problems, such as Alzheimer's and other forms of dementia.

I have never been diagnosed with a mental illness. At times, I have felt depressed or anxious, but it has never reached the point where it affected my day-to-day functioning. Until now.

A Cancer Encounter

I have the unique experience of not only being a mental health professional and helper but also a receiver of services and treatment. My cancer encounter (I don't call it a journey as I prefer to associate this word with pleasant events) was an intensely difficult and physically challenging ordeal due to the harsh treatment regime called the Nigro Protocol (chemotherapy and radiation, also known as chemoradiation).

I was diagnosed with anal cancer (squamous cell carcinoma of the anal canal, stage 3) in May of 2017. My symptoms of frequent, narrow stools, then what I thought were bleeding hemorrhoids, turned out to be a tumor near my butt opening. Not only did I have a tumor, but I also had lymph node involvement. I was put onto a "cancer conveyor belt" of tests including blood tests, a CT scan, an MRI, and a PET scan. To complicate matters, I ended up with a very painful perianal abscess, and I had to go for emergency surgery to clean it out. While in the hospital, I went through a procedure to have a PICC line put into my right arm. This long tube was inserted into my vein so they wouldn't have to poke me every time they wanted a blood sample or to give me chemotherapy.

My cancer treatment started in June. The chemotherapy was given to me via the PICC line, and it included two drugs—Mitomycin-C and fluorouracil (also known as 5-FU). The Mitomycin-C was a purple liquid, and the nurse "pushed it" into my body via a syringe into the PICC line. My husband jokingly referred to it as grape juice. I was provided with a little blue pouch to carry around the chemo pump that would slowly inject the fluorouracil into my body through the PICC line over the next 96 hours. It hung around my neck, and it resembled a baby bottle. The chemical smell was nauseating. I had two rounds of this cocktail; the first was at week one, and the second was at week four.

The pelvic radiation was administered daily, Monday–Friday, for six weeks. It was a 45-minute drive one-way to the hospital. My family and friends helped me get there and back and kept me company. The little tattoos (black dots) on my hips helped the therapists ensure the radiation beams reached the targeted treatment area. I had to ensure my bladder was full. The sessions were quite quick, only about 5–7 minutes long.

Side Effects of Treatment

There are many risks and side effects associated with chemotherapy and radiation. I experienced some of them. Chemotherapy caused me to experience significant fatigue and a "chemo fog," which soon lifted after the pump was taken off. I developed mouth sores, and my hair thinned. I was nauseated and lost my appetite. Overall, I lost 30 pounds.

Radiation caused the most damage. The burns caused by this high-intensity "laser" beam pretty much cooked my pelvic region. As you can imagine, the sensitive lady parts were quite affected, including the waterworks and butt area. I ended up having severe pain. I had tried all kinds of ointments, medications, and even cannabis oil. The burning sensation and "afterburns" (for weeks after treatment) were too much to take sometimes. Having a bowel movement caused me so much pain that I squeezed stress balls to help me cope. One time I called out for Jesus' help, and I dissociated and saw him standing beside me with his white robe and arms outstretched.

My mom had come into town to help me. One particular moment is vivid in my memory. I remember lying in bed in crippling pain. My mom was in bed beside me, and I was holding her hand as I cried and moaned. Having her beside me was better than being alone. My battered, beaten, 51-year-old body was transformed into a vessel of torture I couldn't escape. At that moment, my husband came into the room, and I reached out for his hand as well. Holding their hands, one on each side of me, became a pivotal moment for me. I saw the love and caring in their eyes, their feelings of helplessness, as I sobbed and writhed in pain. I felt the power of their loving support, and I knew if they could have taken my pain away, they would have.

I had to use soaker pads on the bed to catch the seeping fluids and blood that were oozing from my burns. It looked like the aftermath of a battlefield. I took baking soda baths four times a day. I ensured I was keeping hydrated and nourished with fluids and meal supplements. I was told by the dietician to try eating lots of protein.

All the medications, ointments, baths, fluids, nourishment, and appointments for radiation and chemotherapy and other doctors' and specialists' appointments made for a very stressful and busy time. I was consumed with caring for myself, to keep myself clean and ward off infections. I had so much to remember. I prayed a lot. I became overwhelmed with all I had to do, and the pain made everything so much worse. I remember asking my daughter to help me make a chart so I wouldn't forget anything. She helped me figure out a system on a whiteboard that worked.

Hospitalization

At the end of my second round of chemotherapy, I ended up getting a high fever and had to go to the hospital emergency. My heart rate was up to 150 beats per minute, and I was a complete mess. I was shaking and felt like I couldn't cope. I was depressed and overwhelmed. I felt defeated. I desperately wanted to be taken care of.

My burns had reached a peak in terms of pain, and it hurt immensely to urinate and poop. It felt like I was peeing razor blades and pooping cactuses or broken glass. The doctor decided to put in a urinary catheter, and that was a horrible experience in and of itself. I was traumatized. The catheter worked for one night, and then my bladder started to feel full. The nurse did an ultrasound and found my bladder full of urine! "Get this thing out of me!" I thought. She immediately pulled the catheter out. That hurt like hell, too. In hindsight, I wish they had consulted with the radiation oncologist before putting it in. If they had, I wish they had advised against it. I am certain there are other options. I was in such a poor state, feeling wilted and weak. I wasn't able to advocate for myself. I felt injured and had some problems after that (dribbling urine when I stood up, and I was very sore).

Ring the Bell

I was in the hospital for my last radiation treatment, which had been delayed by two days. I was bound and determined to get all 30 treatments done. I was taken by non-urgent stretcher service to another hospital in my hospital gown. I remember early on in my treatments when I was sitting in the waiting room ready to go for my radiation treatment, sometimes people were brought in on stretchers with two orderlies. Now, here I was in the same situation. The good news is that I was able to "ring the bell" to indicate my treatment had ended. I rang that bell long and hard! Although I was weak, I found the strength to make a statement. It was a feeling of accomplishment and hope. When I completed treatment, the staff congratulated me.

The radiation team had warned me that even though the radiation treatments are done, the radiation continues to work for a few weeks after. That's when things got really tough.

Recovery Period (Recovering from Treatment)

After my treatments were completed (August 2, 2017) and I was discharged back home from the hospital a few days later, my healing and recovery period began. I had a lot of physical concerns to attend to, and as I mentioned before, the pain was a big issue. Recovering from treatment is often as big (and sometimes even greater) a deal than the treatment itself.

I noticed a significant decline in the supports once I got home from the hospital. There were no more regular visits to CancerCare Manitoba, and visits to the doctors were fewer and farther between. I found as my skin started to heal, I had less and less routine concerning my self-care. Baths became less frequent. The pain eventually began to subside.

Started to Feel Empty and Lost

I started to feel empty and lost. The person I had been for the past 5-6 months (sick, focused on my treatment and self-care) had less and less of a role. This transition from active treatment to full-time recovery was the hardest. The person I was before the cancer diagnosis was no more either because I was no longer working (on medical leave). I had taken a temporary leave from all my volunteer jobs, and I had stopped most of my regular activities such as shopping, walking the dog, etc.

I discovered I had trouble laughing when I had friends come over to help cheer me up. I had no interests. Nothing made me happy. I tried to watch funny programs, but I found myself just existing. I wanted the time to pass. I had trouble falling asleep; I was up late and slept in. I didn't feel like eating. I had to force myself and remind myself to eat, although I wasn't hungry. I justified not eating by telling myself I was filling up with fluids. I noticed my weight was dropping. I had heard many people lose weight during cancer treatment, so why would I be any different?

I preferred to stay in my pajamas all day. What was the point of getting dressed when I wasn't going anywhere? I wanted to be comfortable. I needed loose-fitting (if any) clothes on my bottom half as I healed. Nighties and long t-shirt style pajamas and a robe were most comfortable. I didn't want to get into the shower; I would have to force myself to wash up. It took too much energy some days. I didn't feel like washing my hair, as I feared it would all fall out (it was thinning and coming out by the handful).

Completely Depleted

Finally, I realized I felt completely depleted. My husband would ask me how I was feeling, and I would say, "Meh." I didn't feel anything. I would sit at the dinner table for a few minutes, very quiet. I would eat a little to appease everyone. My bottom would hurt. I had nothing to say. Then I'd go back upstairs to my bed. I wouldn't want to talk to people on the phone. My text messages were very brief.

Main Concern Was Low Mood

I went to the medical oncologist for a follow-up, and the primary concern at that time was my low mood. He recommended I see my family doctor for this, and he also made a referral to a psychiatrist.

I went to see my family doctor a few days later. I drove myself, which was a big step in getting back to my normal activities. When I saw her, I was a complete mess. I started crying and telling her how hard the last few months had been. By this time, I was convinced I was depressed. I felt completely depleted of any sense of who I was, and I had no interest in much of anything. She asked if I had felt like taking my own life. I said no, but I said I thought it might be nice if I went to sleep and didn't wake up.

I Was Prescribed an Antidepressant

My doctor prescribed an antidepressant and said it wouldn't start to work for a few weeks. I started taking it immediately, and those few weeks were quite difficult. I had friends come by to visit me to help me pass the time. My dog Rocky was my steady companion. My family was busy and would come and go during the day. My friends would send me messages asking how I was doing.

My physical health continued to improve, but my mental health took a dive. My mood was non-existent. I had nothing to do. I had previously cleaned my slate so I could focus on getting better, and once I started to get better, I had a lack of focus.

I Lost Myself

I call this an experience of losing myself. I had to try and find myself again. I had been told by a few others and read that we are never the same after a cancer diagnosis. We end up finding our new normal. Some live in fear of cancer coming back. I've known of people with anal cancer who succumbed to it, so I know there is a real risk of a shortened life.

The irony here is that I have a master's degree in social work, with a graduate specialization in aging. I had imagined living to a ripe old age and using everything I have learned to help myself and others age well. This cancer diagnosis threw me for a loop. I thought, "Isn't that the way it goes? Here I am, an aging specialist who dies of cancer at age 51." It's similar to the unfortunate irony of cancer specialists who die of cancer.

Grief Consumed Me

My sense of loss was profound. My thoughts were consumed with negativity and the anticipated grief of future losses. I'll never get to see my children get married and have children of their own. I won't get to grow old with my husband. I won't get to write my book on

"Aging Well." I felt a huge weight of sadness. Eventually, I must have "numbed out."

I filled my days with watching simple TV programs about animals, veterinarians, and funny home videos. I went on social media and checked out what my friends and family were doing. I watched romantic comedies that I'd seen before.

I Started to Improve

In time, I started to read inspiring books. Eventually, I started writing again. I felt like seeing people. My sleep improved, and I started appreciating food again. I started enjoying my tea and chocolate chip muffins (which was a big clue as to improvement in my mood!).

Within three weeks of being on the antidepressant medication, I was feeling better. My mood improved to the point where I felt good enough to start going out again. I remember going to my friend's house for a couple of hours. That was the start of my venturing out into the real world again. Recovery for me was in baby steps. My mental health slowly returned. My physical health was improving. I had residual physical problems, but those issues were to be worked out in time.

I eventually saw the psychiatrist, and I asked him about my need to continue with the medication, as I was feeling better. He explained based on the description of my symptoms, I had experienced a major depressive episode (MDE). He said there were two explanations for the improvement. One was that the medication helped, and if I went off of it, I would relapse. Two was that I got through my depression on my own. If we go with the second scenario and take me off the medication (slowly), the risk is that I could relapse, and it may not work the second time around. He recommended I stay on the medication for six to nine months. He would send a letter to my family doctor, and she would follow through with his recommendations as she sees fit.

I was relieved to know that I was on the road to recovery, both mentally and physically. I now truly understood what it felt like to be depressed. As a mental health clinician, I had assessed people who were experiencing a clinical depression. Now I had a first-hand account of what it felt like. My family and doctors praised me for getting on it so quickly.

Stigma is Not Helpful

There is a certain amount of stigma surrounding depression. Many times I have heard people say they don't want to take medicine. Based on the literature and research, the best treatment is medication and psychotherapy combined. If people only knew how much medication could help, and that it could be only temporary, maybe they would consider this type of approach to recovery.

There is a certain amount of stigma surrounding not only depression but also anal cancer. I feel I received a double-whammy in this respect. I do not feel the shame like some do, but I know this is indeed in some people's minds. I feel I can put this "behind" me as I continue along this life after a cancer diagnosis.

How I Coped

There were a lot of coping strategies I utilized as I awaited my tests, results, and treatments. One of the first things I did was plant a birch tree in my backyard which I called "The Tree of Hope." I also bought a stuffed lamb, which I named Hope. Here's a list of other things that helped me pass the time and offered me something to focus on (in no particular order):

- ✓ adult coloring books
- ✓ crosswords
- ✓ prayer
- ✓ church (Sunday mass, Novena mass)
- ✓ movies
- ✓ TV (recorded some light programs, those about animals were especially comforting)
- ✓ sitting outside in nature, especially by bodies of water
- ✓ walks outside
- ✓ funny programs (e.g., America's Funniest Home Videos)
- ✓ reading
- ✓ writing
- ✓ journaling my feelings and thoughts

- ✓ surfing the Internet
- ✓ listening to music
- ✓ cuddling with my dog
- ✓ visiting with friends
- ✓ talking to a psychologist/friend
- ✓ emails/texting
- ✓ playing games on my cell phone
- ✓ meditation and mindfulness
- ✓ online support group

What I did not find helpful:

- the news
- too much responsibility
- eating in bed, alone

The news (in 2017) was full of horrible tragedies, natural disasters, political unrest in the USA, and other situations beyond my control. There were no positive or uplifting messages to gain by consuming myself with the current events of the day. I eventually stopped listening to and watching the news.

I found if I had too many things to be responsible for, it tended to muddle my mind. At times I just wanted other people to look after me. Medications, ointments, personal care tasks, eating healthy (asking for food and drink when I was bedridden), etc. was too much for me to handle sometimes. At one point the dietician told my family to " . . . just put the food beside her bed. If she eats it, or some of it, that's great."

Holistic Approach to Healing and Recovery

Overall, a holistic body, mind, and spirit approach to wellness helped me get through the six-month ordeal. I looked after my body as well as I could with the help and recommendations from the healthcare professionals and my family. I looked after my mind by keeping it active and stimulated to a level that was not too much and not too little.

For example, I tried to watch some movies that were too stimulating and fast-paced, so I had to turn them off. I cared for my spirit by listening to my need to get closer to God and be true to myself. I wasn't able to give as much as I had given of myself in the past, and I had to learn how to accept and receive. I received and believed in all the loving, powerful, positive prayers, and good wishes I received from my family and friends. I maintained hope. I believed "this too shall pass."

Ways to Nurture and Stimulate Through Our Senses

The only way we have access into our body and mind is through our five senses. Some believe in our sixth sense of intuition. Here are some ways to nurture and entertain yourself:

- o **Hearing:** Music, audio books, white noise, nature sounds, self-affirmations
- o **Sight:** Nice photos, videos, scenery, colors, nature, inspirational quotes, car rides, walks, museums
- o **Touch:** Cozy blankets, socks, shawls, fan blowing, shopping (touch new things)

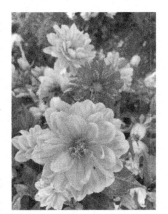

- o **Smell:** Essential oils, favorite foods, flowers, outdoors (Essential oils are another way to help calm the mind, especially lavender essential oil.)
- o **Taste:** Favorite foods, drinks, lozenges, gum
- o **Intuition:** Knowing or sensing based on feelings versus facts. In other words, "trusting your gut" or "having a hunch."

Communication and Self-Expression

I stayed connected to my closest family and friends by writing a private online blog. I posted my concerns, my progress, and my setbacks. This way I didn't have to repeat myself every time I saw them or spoke to them. We were able to focus on other things when we talked or got together. I also wrote my innermost fears and concerns in a private journal. I spoke to a social worker, a priest, and a psychologist. I shared my feelings with my husband, my mother, and my closest friends.

The Importance of Mental Health

My cancer encounter and post-treatment ordeal taught me a lot about depression, pain, taking things one day at a time, and the importance of connecting with others. Mental health is as important as physical health. If you are not healthy mentally, there is no way you are going to have much ability to cope with the physical problems that come your way. It also helped me learn to imagine some of those sad and low moments in our lives like a bad weather system—they eventually pass.

If you ever find yourself like me, having a disrupted sleep schedule, struggling to get up, get washed and dressed, feeling numb, avoiding social interaction, losing weight, and finding it difficult to text more than a couple of words, it's essential to seek professional help. There are many other symptoms of depression such as feelings of worthlessness, suicidal thoughts, and agitation. Some of us can't get through it alone. You're worth it.

****

RESOURCE:

Mayo Clinic. "Depression (major depressive disorder)." Retrieved 03 Sep 2018. https://www.mayoclinic.org/diseases-conditions/depression/symptoms-causes/syc-20356007

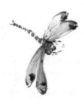

Chapter 7

Journal Notes—On Sexuality, Relationships, and Anxiety

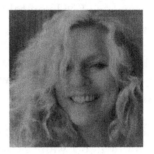

Sharie Vance

I journal. I have done it for years. Sometimes, I go back and read what I wrote, and I am amazed by what my younger self was afraid of or thought was important. After my cancer treatment was over and I got busy again, I felt it was necessary to move on.

I wonder now if I should have remained connected to my survivor friends. After losing a few of them to metastasis, I think I distanced myself because I was scared. I never mention the fear after I had my port removed only a week after my treatment ended. I rarely mention cancer in my entries either.

It is clear I have had a great deal of anxiety and self-doubt. I struggled with sexuality issues and relationships. In retrospect, perhaps this was caused by the trauma of treatment—and not talking to survivors. I'm not sure. When I was diagnosed, I had just finished my 2nd year of graduate school. Graduate school is humbling enough—graduate school and cancer —well, it was a lot.

Have a peek into my journal over a span of 4.5 years. You'll learn about some of the men in my life, my anxieties and fears, my struggles (and triumphs) with sexuality, my work, and my passion. You may be able to relate to some of it; other parts may offer you some insight into my internal conflict. It starts with an entry prior to the cancer diagnosis and ends with some questions about the future.

Sharie's Journal

<u>July 20, 2013</u>. The idea of accepting I am all that I will ever be saddens me. Why? Is it because I've been told all my life to want to be more? Maybe it is because we all tell each other never to settle—be who you want to be—have what it is you want to have—and that is the problem. You must know what it is you want to be and what it is you want to have. What I have is not awful, so why am I not content to accept it is the best I can do?

I want the freedom to do whatever it is I want to do. But I also want the freedom to help others when I want to help them. The pain of not being able to support my family when they need me—either to pay a bill or to help them go to school or even to fly them or myself so that we can be together is excruciating.

I think it is so painful because I believe it is the only way I can be of use to my children. I do not want them to have to bear the burden of me. I just need to focus on what I can do to become a better friend to them.

Why do I now insist on living a life that does not make me happy? Can I even be happy? I need to focus on what does make me happy and let go of things I think might make me happy but destroy my relationships from inattention.

I feel like it is time for a radical change in how I see my life and the way I approach it. I have been pushing myself and making excuses for myself for far too long. What if I do have cancer? When it really comes down to it, will I regret all my decisions? Which ones will I not? What will I wish I had done or not done?

August 4, 2013. I've given myself permission today to wallow in unproductiveness. I mean seriously, I may find out tomorrow I have cancer. I can't go too far away from the toilet, and I really can't make any plans until I know one way or the other, so why bother being productive? How about I just relax and enjoy myself?

This medication really works. I'm shitting water. No cramps. No feelings of pressure at all. There is just a sudden, unshakable certainty the contents of my bowels will be all over me if I don't get to a toilet ASAP.

Getting a Diagnosis Changed my Life

August 5, 2013. My life changed today. Completely and irrevocably changed. I'm glad I gave myself permission to relax yesterday. However, it is odd how calm I feel now, considering. Pretty soon I could be wearing a colostomy bag. That is one of the most disgusting things I can think of—a shit bag hanging from my side. But, that is something I will deal with if I have to—I mean, think about it—a shit bag is better than dying.

The way I see my family and especially Tony changed today, too. Whatever barriers I have placed in the way of accepting their love for me have changed. I see things clearly now.

August 8, 2013. Got the call Tuesday evening. No shit bag! But, I have cancer. Anal cancer to be exact. Chemo and radiation are the treatments. So not looking forward to that! I am wishing now I had not procrastinated on so many things . . . my thesis proposal, editing my movie, moving in with Tony—agh! The list is so long! Of course, NOW I'm paralyzed by how much I need to get done before my treatments start.

August 12, 2013. I have an appointment with the oncologist tomorrow. I'm so angry I could scream. This was not supposed to happen!!! I'm about to be subjected to poison and radiation to kill what will kill me if I don't. I HATE THIS!!!!!!! I am furious at the possible wasted potential that is me. I know there is so much more I could have done with my life if I just wasn't scared to try. Should I make promises to a deity I don't believe in? Should I say I will try if I get out of this alive?

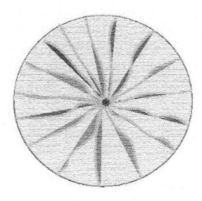

Figure 2. Sharie's depiction of an anus.

A Call to Arms

August 13, 2013. I've been in a funk for days—withdrawn, snappish, depressed. My weekend with Tony was not a good one. We didn't fight, but I just didn't want to be there. I wanted to be alone.

We spend our weekdays living 40 miles apart. We've conducted our relationship like this for years, and it's worked, but we've known for a while it is well past time to join households. I've chickened out on him three times over the years, but October 1st is the date. We are moving in together.

And now this. All day today I've fought sudden tears and the gravity of self-pity. But it wasn't until one of my friends called me did I realize that the emotion really responsible for my funk was not sadness, but anger—really deep anger cloaked in the shadow of depression. Barb is a research coordinator at a cancer research hospital, but she's never had cancer, so her "everything will be okay" and "just keep a positive attitude" made me want to scream. I'm terrified. I'm stuck on underground tracks, and the light in front of me is not the end of the tunnel but a fucking train! Don't pat me on the head and say keep a positive attitude! Fortunately, I didn't say that to her. She's one of my best friends, and she means well.

When I got off the phone, I went for a drive. I haven't eaten much today and thought I'd grab something to go. Not being hungry means I drove a long time. On my way home, Tony called, but I didn't want to talk. He seemed annoyed with me when I hung up. Who the hell does he think he is? I have a right to be bitchy. I have fucking cancer. I gnawed on that one while I walked the dog. He's going to make my recovery hard. It's going to be all about him, and I'm going to have to take care of him instead of the other way around. Maybe I shouldn't move in with him. Maybe I should just call the whole thing off!

A few hours later he tries again. By now, I'm feeling a little less angry and a little more needing a shoulder. He said, "I'll be your punching bag." So I let him have it—my anger and my terror. I'm living a real-life horror movie here! Things aren't supposed to be like this! I sobbed and blew my way through half a roll of toilet paper.

He said, "Your feelings are perfectly understandable. And those around you are feeling things too. You know what keeps me from being terrified? My faith . . . in you. I have 100% faith in you. Give it a few days for things to sink in . . . I know you . . . you love a good challenge. You'll see this as just one more thing you have overcome. You are a fighter—a tough girl. You'll beat this. I'm absolutely positive, and that's what keeps me from being terrified. Once everything has settled in and you get your mind right, you'll do what you need to do."

I swear I could hear music and see a flag waving in the background as I pictured him pacing back and forth rallying the troops. My very own General Patton was giving me a "Call to Arms!"

"Aye! Aye! Captain!" I said, pride swelling my chest. He's right. I'm a fighter, and I can do this, especially because he's in my corner. I'm a lucky girl . . . maybe I'll move in with him after all.

Editor's note: Original post: youcaring.com/medical-fundraiser/sharie-vance-s-cancer-fight/79277 (Posted August 16, 2013).

Treatment

<u>September 3, 2013</u>. First day of treatment—woke up with a cold sore on my lip. Stress probably. Tony drove up from Dallas to be with

me. Received an injection (infusion?) of mitomycin, then was suited up with a mechanical pump, a bag of 5-FU, and an ugly, poorly designed fanny pack. Tony napped with me all day. Got a "care" package from my daughter. Contained art supplies, dry mouth lozenges, tea for digestion, Eucerin lotion, aloe vera socks (my grandson picked them out), lip balm, and an awesome snuggly blanket. The card made me cry.

September 5, 2013. Lots of nausea, no vomiting, very tired—which could have been caused by the antinausea meds that I took regularly. I basically slept my way through the first two days. I had an overall sensation of just not feeling well—"jack nasty" as my blogger friend, Michelle, aptly named it. After that, although I couldn't eat much, the nausea went away.

September 7, 2013. Woke up feeling extremely weak and dreamlike. Perhaps I had overdone things, or the radiation had started affecting me. The pump was removed. Drove to Dallas to be with Tony. It took me two hours to get ready (normally takes me 15 minutes). Felt like I was walking underwater. Noticed a sore throat and bleeding gums (while brushing) later that night. Had developed a sore "spot" on the right side of my throat. (Have been using salt/soda water to rinse my mouth out. Hopefully, that will keep things under control.)

September 8, 2013. More energy. Appetite returned somewhat, but NOTHING tasted good. :(Cramping, but no diarrhea.

September 9, 2013. Busy day! Spent morning at the clinic—I've lost 9 lbs.! I need to lose 35, so I'm not complaining. Saw both oncologists and had blood drawn. White blood count (WBC) already a little on the low side. Got a flu shot. Talked to the financial counselor (cancer is expensive). Was starving by the time I left. Stopped for a biscuit and got a waffle/egg/sausage thing instead— HUGE mistake. Could only eat half. Paid for it later. Went to work for 3.5 hours, left because of cramping. Got home just in time!

September 10, 2013. Woke up with two more cold sores, but otherwise feeling like a normal human being. Went to class and also instructed lab. No cramping. Yay! Drove to radiation, came home and took a nap. Woke up feeling kind of weak and having some cramping, but I'm better now.

Since I feel okay right now—I'm writing this blog and trying to catch up on a few organizational things I can do to make my life easier. Fall semester is in full swing, and we are moving at the end of the month. There's no time to be sick, dammit!

I actually feel like a failure for having cancer. I also have a fear of failure regarding my side effects and my ability to work and go to school. I'm already doubting my ability to "handle" it all. That makes me feel like a failure too. I feel like I'm going to do the wrong things; I'm not going to take care of myself well enough, and I won't ask for help until it's too late.

Six Months After Diagnosis—Getting Nowhere

March 5, 2014. I have so many things to do, and yet I do none of them. Don't want to really. Doesn't interest me. What does? Feeling sorry for myself. Thinking about doing things rather than doing them. Wondering why my life isn't better. Am I holding myself back? Is Tony holding me back? Does my inability to do the work mean I don't want to do it, or am I just scared to try? I do seem to have a lot of fear. Fear of the future mostly, but there are others.

So, to feel better for not doing all or any of the multiple things I desperately need to be doing, things that would prove my vocation choice if I'd just do them, I am writing this down. Maybe writing it down will help me.

March 10, 2014. Riding behind everything is the fear I'm running out of time. Longevity is no longer guaranteed. I can no longer claim youth's blissful ignorance of the truth. When you are young, you think you will live forever, or at least until you are very old. Becoming old happens in some misty, faraway future—nothing to worry about in the immediacy of being young. But then you find out you are not bulletproof. You are vulnerable. You will die. Your time is finite.

Hopeful But Anxious

<u>July 28, 2014</u>. I am beginning to feel hope again for the first time in a long time. I have to trust my instincts artistically and stop second-guessing myself. I've been looking at footage as well as painting and reading old notes I've written. It's not my talent I doubt; it's my willingness to work as hard as I need to in order to make something happen. Finishing the Kickstarter video and getting mostly positive feedback has a lot to do with this renewed sense of hope. It felt so good to finish something. It means I'm making progress. Finally.

It's a frightening thing, my life. Most of the time, I feel like I'm on the edge of the planet and I'm about to fall off. Spin off into nothingness. A relief from this constant anxiety I feel. I don't think this is normal at all. That's why the hope feels so good. Maybe I'm not drowning. Maybe I'll be okay.

<u>August 21, 2014</u>. Have been stressing a lot lately. Are bad moods habitual? I mean, can I always be unhappy as a habit rather than a fact? You know, like there really isn't anything wrong with my life, I am unhappy because I don't know how to be happy? Interesting thought.

I keep reminding myself of that each time I feel those familiar butterflies. These butterflies are not the sweet, being around someone you like butterflies. Nor are these butterflies the ones that attack at the precipice of a roller coaster. These butterflies have fangs. Big fangs that dig into my stomach and suck the joy out of everything. That's what I call anxiety. That feeling right there. I wonder if it's habitual, too.

Unnamed Tension Builds

<u>September 21, 2014</u>. Rarely do we speak without being defensive with each other. It's like we need a good fight. There is tension underneath that doesn't seem to have a name. I wanted to take a nap, and the TV was on; it bothers me, so I leave. He wants me to return—he's turned it off. He thinks I'm mad because it was on. I'm mad because I don't have a space I can go to when I want to lie down without having to tell him to turn it off. I'm not sure that makes sense. Maybe I'm mad because I have to share the room.

September 29, 2014. Telling someone personal things, i.e., I'm a filmmaker = Wrong. "Why would you tell someone you don't know personal stuff?" Seriously? Cooking a meatloaf for someone coming over, because I know he likes my meatloaf, and I enjoy his company = Wrong. Going out with the girls = Wrong (because I will drink or perhaps some male will look at me.) Drinking when we are out together = Wrong. Drinking period = Wrong. It makes me want to drink just to be rebellious.

I wish I could tell him just how stupid, disgusting, and boring I sometimes think he is. The only right thing about our relationship is the comfort I feel when I snuggle up to him or when he tells me I can do something I'm afraid I can't do. He's not abusive, and he gives me the agreed upon amount of money each month, so I'm not stuck paying for everything.

Pretty much everything else sucks. Ok—maybe "sucks" is too harsh. Here's the deal: I've become fat and lazy and isolated, and much of the time, I blame him for that. I know some of this is because I'm busy with work, which requires me to sit at a computer a lot. Some of that computer time is, of course, me on Facebook.

So, I do my thing, and he does his, and I'm lonely as hell. I want people I can talk to!!! People I can hang out with, discuss art and liberal politics. Honestly, I'm bored as fuck (and there's none of that going on either). Unfortunately, I feel restricted even to seek out new friendships—male or female. I don't like to feel restricted.

Addendum: My dear, late friend, Barb hardly recognized me when I finally had a chance to visit her in January 2015. It wasn't until she asked me "What the hell is wrong with you?" did I realize I had been grieving the loss of my sexuality. I broke down and cried. Afterwards, she made me promise to seek help, and I did.

Lost My Sexy

Preamble: After undergoing radiation treatment for anal cancer, I did not have complete control over my bladder. I would wear those very thin panty liners for almost a year afterward. Additionally, I was never certain if I had full control over my rectum. I was always afraid of being "dirty." This meant sexually I became very inhibited. I wouldn't allow my partner Tony to touch me unless I first made sure I was completely clean. Not that he wanted to touch me often.

Once I was diagnosed, it seemed he lost all interest. He certainly wasn't interested in helping me with the vaginal dilators or talking about it or much of anything regarding sex or romance. I was quite miserable. So much so that almost a year after I was pronounced no evidence of disease (NED), I had fallen into a terrible depression, gained 30 pounds, and stopped taking care of myself. All I had energy for was my thesis.

<u>March 21, 2015</u>. "So I'm like on this crazy hormone regime," I say as I am walking out of the closet. He's in his usual evening position. On the bed. Watching TV. "I'm on a patch (pulling up my shirt and pointing at the tiny plastic dot on my pudgy stomach). I am taking progesterone by mouth. I haven't had progesterone since I don't know when." He continues to stare at the TV. "Ovaries make three hormones; estrogen, progesterone and testosterone. I've only ever been on estrogen and testosterone. Anyway, the third thing is an estrogen tablet I break in half and put up inside my vagina."

This gets his attention. Briefly. He scowls, but his eyes return to the TV. The scowl remains on his face. "Every Monday, Wednesday, and Friday. It's not unheard of . . . I mean, I've heard of it, so it's not weird. He feels sure he can fix it." Eyes on TV. Scowl is gone. "He also thinks it'll fix my leaky bladder problem, too. I mean, it's a lot better than it used to be, but still. He said estrogen makes the urethra sticky." Eyes on the TV.

"I can tell you are just fascinated by this amazing chemistry stuff." I'm laughing as I walk around the bed watching him watch TV. "I guess all you need to take away from this is that one day we can have sex again." He looks at me but says nothing. "Well, maybe," I say as I'm walking into the bathroom. "I can tell you are just thrilled about that." I shut the door.

"What the hell is that supposed to mean?" I hear from the other side. "I'm just trying to watch a movie here."

The next day, he wants to talk about something unusual he's seen on the drive home. I stare right at him. Half smile and walk away from him when he's finished. "What's wrong with you?" he asks from his usual reclining position.

I'm halfway down the hall when I yell back, "Nothing."

"Oh come on! Don't do this," I hear as I make my way to the kitchen. I'm not doing anything. My heart pounds. I walk back to my office. The front door creaks as he returns from his cigarette break. I pick up a highlighter and pretend to read the sentence in front of me. He comes into my office and shuts the door. Crap.

When I'm emotional, I don't remember exact words as much as I do exact feelings. He apologized. He's not very communicative. We don't know if the treatment will work—if it does, yay! It's not a big deal. Blah blah blah. I tell him I no longer feel sexy.

He counters with something about the treatment for my type of cancer. I feel ugly. He says, "Oh, come on. You know you are not." This makes me angry.

"Maybe I need you to tell me I am attractive."

"That's not what I do," he says. "You catch me looking at your butt, and then you have to ask me about it."

"Because I want to hear you tell me."

"But I like to play the game."

"Right. I'm telling you I need more than your game. I need you to tell me." I think it ended in a stalemate. He hugged me at some point, although I kind of suspect he wanted to see if I had been drinking, but maybe not. He never did tell me I'm attractive.

A Fake Relationship

March 28, 2015. The thing is, you can tell when you are not getting 100% of a person. It's just not there. When you doubt yourself so much that you don't believe what you are seeing, when you don't believe what you are feeling, you have lost yourself. It isn't the other person's fault, though, that you have.

You wanted to believe he was a sweet, wonderful, honest guy, but you never quite could, and you stayed anyway. I vow to myself right now that I will never again do this to myself. I will never again talk myself into a relationship. Ever. I am done torturing others and myself with my relationship woes. It's ridiculous.

I hated the thought that the something I need to do is break up with Tony. But every time I've had the perfect excuse, I've always gone back to him. I will have to do the work of figuring it out later. Or perhaps I won't. I think a review of my journals will show I have tried to figure this out for years, and here I am—still with him.

What am I worth? What does it say about how I view myself by staying with him? It says that I'm okay with being second best. He's second best to me, after all. I mean, I put my own agenda ahead of him. We never speak of sex or kissing. I flirt with other guys. I just flirt, though, and not even sexually. I am not even sure I'd call it flirting.

He never bothers me. He's here. He doesn't make demands. But he's restrictive in a way I can't describe. And I'm terribly unhappy with our sex life, even before I had cancer. Terribly unhappy. But I never talked about it. Well, I tried; I just didn't do a very good job of it.

So why am I with him? Because when he does pay attention to me, in the way that I want him to, which is pretty much never, but still, when he did, I am jelly. But that would always go away, and he'd go back to being the emotionally unavailable (to me) person that he is.

We both have our faults. But what am I worth in the eyes of other people when I stay with someone I obviously hold in contempt? What does that tell the people I admire about me? It says I don't love myself as I should. And now. Now I know he considers this relationship fake. He's not happy, either. He'll lie of course and say he is. He's a survivor.

Anyway. I have to break up with him. Today. When he comes home. I refuse to play the game anymore. Standing up for myself is terrifying. I'm shaking at the thought of our confrontation. Here's hoping I don't chicken out.

<u>March 29, 2015</u>. I didn't chicken out. I don't think I've ever been prouder of myself. :)

I Should Have Said Something

Preamble: I gave myself a couple of months and then started dating again. An old acquaintance—someone who had pursued me during one of my many breaks with Tony, came around, and I took him up on his offer.

<u>June 28, 2015</u>. I think I should have been more honest with him—told him it hurt—told him to slow down—told him it wasn't okay—told him I needed more time, and it was not okay that we had just fucked for an hour, and now we were leaving the hotel room, and I'm bleeding, and I didn't get off.

For crying out loud. He didn't try to warm me up first. He just went to it. There was no foreplay, and once he was done, he was done. I had given him permission to orgasm. I had told him it was okay. So now why am I ready to not ever see him again?

I know I built it up in my head. It was going to be so fantastic. And it could have been, but it wasn't. It wasn't good at all. I lay there thinking, why don't I say something? I was mute. I couldn't even speak of mundane things. All I could think about was "how disappointing." It reminded me of the beginning of my relationship with Tony when I let him get away with all sorts of things I couldn't later backtrack on. Things that caused a lot of resentment.

When we text—I told him I should have said something. He said I did, but he couldn't stop. Sorry! I'm sorry, too, I told him. If that's the case, and the results are pain, blood, and more medical bills, I fail to see what my incentive is to continue doing it. And that was that.

Sexuality and Its Effect on Creativity

<u>August 16, 2015</u>. This whole film, *Miz Markley & Me*, is a statement of the fact that I achieved what I set out to do: make a music video of "Eve Takes the Fall," highlight Lisa's talents, and offer a different view of the world of female artists of a certain look and age that's largely absent in broadcast media.

I did a lot more, too. I uncovered the literature regarding women in the world of music, the cultural reflection of popular female music, and theories of image and female sexuality and how it connected to the story I had created from Lisa's life and music.

It did not connect until I read *Vagina, A New Biography* by Naomi Wolf. Then everything made sense. Naomi's research uncovered the connection between healthy sexuality and the effects damaged sexuality can have on an artist's ability to create. Bruce turned Lisa on, and she went for it. What's more feminist than that? Look at her life. She's the most creative person I know. She radiates creativity, and she's very much in charge of her life, even when she leans on Bruce. Their relationship is definitely sexual, and as evident from their behavior toward each other, it's a mutually satisfying one.

Singer/Songwriter Gina Forsyth is much kinder and gentler from having good sex in her life. She is a genius on the fiddle and is asked to play all over the United States and Europe. Women who understand the importance of good sex can appreciate a woman's courage for leaving a sexually devoid relationship to be with someone who gives her lovely orgasms. It's okay to be sexual. It's okay to be happy.

Two Souls

<u>November 15, 2015</u>. I believe in a creative source. But I don't see it as an entity. I see it as a phenomenon. It is something outside my comprehension.

I feel the pull of Don's soul toward mine. It complicates things that I don't believe in souls—at least not on the metaphysical plane—or at least I didn't think I did until just now. Maybe we do have souls— at least while we are living. A conscientiousness that resonates and can feel in tune with something else. Something that resonates on the same frequency perhaps.

One Thought Changes it All

December 31, 2015. Goodness. It's been a busy year. It's been a bizarre, strange, sometimes very sad, and wonderful year. I have no jobs lined up. I have no idea what I'm going to do for money. I should be terrified. But I'm not. This past year taught me a lot of things. Make time for my family and friends. Ask for help. Losing weight can be done. I am capable. I don't hate my life anymore. I'm actually pretty excited.

Last year I was so miserable. I had no idea what would happen. Over the past year, I was fortunate enough to have opportunities I could take advantage of, but I had to take the steps necessary to make them happen. And it took one thought to give me the motivation: "I'm worthy."

That may not sound like much, or it may even sound cheesy and trite, but it's everything, really. This thought did not necessarily resonate with me. Many people, including my kids and friends, helped me believe that.

Anxiety No More

January 25, 2016. Okay—I re-read a lot of old journal entries. It seems I pondered philosophical questions about being human more than I do now. I also worried constantly about my relationship with Tony and had a great deal of anxiety about not only my future but also my choice of occupation—actually, a great deal of anxiety over most of my decisions.

It's good not to have that constant worry. I can't say why I no longer have it. A quick guess is that I have proven to myself that it's all good. I'll be okay. Perhaps it is because I'm away from that relationship now, and I've decided I love production design (specifically location scouting and set decorating/prop finding) Maybe it's because I have a job, even if it's temporary. Maybe it's because I have Don.

Oh, the Terror

July 27, 2016. I waste so much time thinking. I'm not even sure what I think about all day. I just know I don't seem to get a lot done. I read a lot. Too much, I think. I keep trying to absorb information, but I don't seem to be able to. I almost let my medication run out. I don't want to talk to anybody. At least not really. I do, but I don't. I don't feel as if I have anything useful to say.

Sometimes I feel like I'm holding on by my fingernails. I don't know how to stop the terror I live with every day. What's my terror? What could I possibly be afraid of besides getting old and dying in poverty, painfully and unloved? Or even worse, watching my kids die? I live in terror that I really am nothing. Or that I'm something, but I am too lazy to make anything out of it. I think I'm stupid. I think I don't know anything. I don't think I am fit to teach because, like Jon Snow, I know nothing.

Addendum: Eight months later.

March 1, 2017. Today, I met Don at the jewelry store. I found my ring. It is very sparkly. I love my ring. He puts a deposit on the ring, and we go out to eat. We talk about wedding plans. Should we get a cover band or let an original band play? I want to get married around 6 pm because it's beautiful lighting.

Trish is at my house for 5 hours. When she leaves, my hair is noticeably blonder and 4 inches shorter. I like it. Don likes it. Everyone is happy. Life is good.

Much to Be Thankful For—Including Sex

May 1, 2017. I do a lot of thinking and worrying these days. I have nothing to complain about. I have a wonderful guy. I love him. He loves me. I can live with him. We have wonderful sex. I have a great job that I am not really sure I can do, or if I really want to, but it is the job I said I was going to have a long time ago. I live in a great house, and I get to go on vacations. I am fairly healthy. My family and friends are all fairly happy and healthy (even if some are dealing with personal dramas, they won't prove fatal, I hope). I don't live in a war zone. I have much to be thankful for.

June 1, 2017. We got married yesterday. He called me "Mrs." this morning, and I giggled. This is something I set out to do: marry an intelligent, educated, attractive, well-off man who adores me (especially when I cook him dinners and work out with him.) Someone I could make a home with. Someone I could fuss over, and he could spoil me. Someone to have great sex with.

I married a wonderful guy. He likes to take me places. And he is generous with my family. I married well. This is an accomplishment.

January 15, 2018. I wonder what I'll be writing about next year at this time, my success or my failure? Do I get to keep my job? Do I become an awesome teacher? Does this shit finally make sense to me? Have I done anything good? Is everyone okay? Am I okay?

The future is funny. A great place to imagine—but the present never looks like the future imagined. Sometimes it's better, and sometimes it's worse, but rarely is it precisely the way you figured (if you figured at all.)

✸✸✸✸✸✸✸✸✸✸

RESOURCE:

Sharie's Blog–Anal Cancer: Anus Funny as You Think (*anusfunnyasyouthink.com*)

Chapter 8

My Abdominoperineal Resection and Colostomy Story

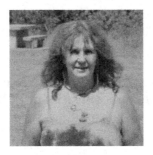

Joy Anderson

Four years ago (when I was 58), I was diagnosed with stage 3 anal cancer, with metastasis to the lymph nodes. I went through a combination of radiation and chemotherapy (chemo), which took care of the lymph nodes. Since the cancer was still there, even though it had shrunk some, they wanted to do an abdominoperineal resection (APR). This involves removing the anus and possibly other body parts. Needless to say, this scared me.

I looked up online what the APR involved and sent a note to my radiologist. The radiologist suggested brachytherapy (the insertion of radioactive implants directly into or near the tumor), which I also went through. Looking back, I should have skipped brachytherapy, as anal probes are not my fetish. But telling the doctors that can be fun.

Scheduled for APR Surgery

Unfortunately after all this radiation, the cancer was still there and trying to come back with a vengeance. I was scheduled to have the APR. I was also told they were going to remove my uterus and ovaries due to how much radiation they had been exposed to and the possibility of another cancer coming as a result.

I did a lot of research to educate myself about what I was about to undergo. I asked the doctors and ostomy nurses a lot of questions. The American Cancer Society website (*cancer.org*) has useful information on different types of surgeries for the treatment of cancer. I didn't stick with just one resource though; I did Internet searches on anal cancer, the APR, living with an ostomy, etc. Always look for more than one source. There is a lot of misleading info out there. However, I find if the same thing is repeated, it's usually good info.

I went in for the APR surgery expecting it to be only a few hours—it lasted 12. They ended up removing a lot more than initially planned. The doctors were great at making sure my family was kept informed.

Part of the procedure was called a flap, where they took the tissue out of my leg (it was going to be either my leg or stomach), and it was turned inside my body to fill in the holes where the anus and surrounding tissue used to be. With this, you gain what a lot of us call a "Barbie or Ken Butt." Your butt looks normal, but no longer has a hole.

It is kind of strange to think that skin that was on my thigh is now on my butt. The surgeon had to take more out of my leg than expected due to how much was removed, and now I walk with a limp. I was warned that this might happen.

Another part of the surgery was receiving a colostomy because to get rid of the cancer they had to remove my anus ("Barbie Butt"). I had looked into getting an artificial anus, yes, there are some, but all require that you still have something to attach it to. Also, there are a lot of issues dealing with these.

For those of you who don't know, a colostomy is where they take the end of your intestine and pull it out through a hole in your abdomen. This opening is called a stoma. A bag (also called a pouch or ostomy appliance) is attached to catch the waste. It really isn't as bad as it sounds, and to be honest, it was kind of a relief not having to use the bedpan while I was recovering. Changing and cleaning a bag was a lot easier.

When I first got out of surgery, they had me on a morphine pump. I was to press a button every so many minutes for pain control. I am not a big fan of pain meds, and I guess my tolerance for medication is low. I was having some really weird dreams. They were mostly about the ostomy bag falling off.

My pain was mostly from muscle spasms and acid reflux, and the morphine wasn't helping with it. They were only letting me have liquids until my bowels started working. A liquid diet was causing the acid reflux, and, guess what, the morphine can cause constipation. Since the morphine wasn't helping, I decided to stop taking it. Everything started working.

The pain from the actual surgery wasn't all that bad. The next day the nurse came to tell me they were weaning me off the morphine. She was surprised when I informed her it was not necessary as I had already done so myself!

Recovery and Rehabilitation

I got another surprise when the plastic surgeon told me I could not bend at the waist for six weeks, and I was only allowed to sit up at a 20° angle. I only expected to be in the hospital for a few days. Try getting out of bed without bending at the waist—and do you truly understand just how little a 20° angle is? This was to keep the flap from tearing loose from where it was still attached, keeping a blood flow to the area.

It was interesting how they would get me up to walk. They would tilt the bed, and I would roll off with a nurse to help me. We did the reverse for getting me back in. This created a problem for me going home. It was arranged for me to go to a Veterans Affairs (VA) rehabilitation (rehab) facility. I spent almost three weeks in the hospital and the rest of the six weeks in the rehab facility.

One funny thing with all this while I was in the hospital, I was supposed to walk at least once every day. The physical therapy people weren't able to come daily, so the nurses had to help. The plastic surgeon was upset because they were not getting me up to walk. I asked him if he had seen the size of the nurses. I am not a small woman, 5'10", and at that time weighed almost 200 lbs. The nurses were these little twiggy things—I doubt they were 100 pounds soaking wet. He laughed and helped get me over to the rehab facility faster.

Even at the rehab facility, they had "fun" with me. "You can't bend at the waist? You are only allowed to bend 20°? How do we get you up?" I had to show them how it worked. I was also doing what I could in the bed. Just rolling from side to side was a chore, but by doing so, I didn't have to use the very uncomfortable wedges that help prevent bedsores. The plastic surgeon let me know how high I could raise my legs, and I was doing that as well. When the physical therapy people saw what I was doing, they left me alone. I was amazed at how weak I was after the surgery.

They have hand-held female urinals, which are much easier than the bedpan. The bedpan actually caused me issues as some of the stitches on my bottom pulled loose. For about five weeks, the nurses had to pack that area until it healed.

I was excited when the doctor finally let me sit up. That was about the same time I was able to walk with a cane instead of a walker. It felt good to be able to walk out of the rehab facility.

I was blessed during this time by having family and friends coming by and visiting with me. My daughter stayed up at the rehab facility for the first few days. My boyfriend of 17 years was there every weekend. He brought me my Kindle and computer. I detest watching TV; I jokingly say it kills brain cells.

The facility let my family bring me what I normally eat for breakfast instead of what they served. I would typically eat a bowl of granola cereal with almond milk. They even kept the almond milk in the fridge for me. I had a little problem getting the dietician to understand that I have an allergy to artificial sweeteners, but after my daughter sent them a few notes asking if they were trying to poison her mother, it got straightened out.

During all this time, the ostomy nurse would come to see me once a week and check on my progress of adapting to having a colostomy. I am so glad I looked up all the YouTube videos on this. Kudos to those folks willing to do this. It helped a lot. I really believe doing all this helped me to accept the fact I will wear a bag for life. I got to see, beforehand, that there are very few limitations just because I wear a bag. I have been back to the gym, swimming, boating, and doing my best to enjoy life. I did have a doctor give me a heads-up to be careful with using my abdominal muscles as I basically have a medically-induced hernia. That means I have to be careful how much weight I lift. I use this as an excuse to get the guys to carry in any heavy animal food sacks and bales of hay as I live on a small farm and used to do this myself.

I did have to change types and brands on the ostomy bags. On the first change, it was from a two-piece to a one-piece. The two-piece has a kind of plate you put on first that the bag attaches to. This made it easier to put on. But as I became more active, I found this to be bulky, and it affected what bending I could do. It was an ostomy nurse who suggested the one-piece.

Also with getting more active, I had some trouble with "blowouts" and decided to check out some of the free samples other companies offer. Once I found one that worked for me, it was easy getting my prescription changed through the ostomy nurse. It is not a bad idea to check with the companies who carry ostomy supplies for samples every so often. Not only does it let you know what is available, but it gives you extras if you need them.

So far, going through VA, they have been good at supplying what I need. I do have to give them almost a month to refill my prescription, but they send me at least a three-month supply—three boxes of 10 bags each. I usually order more about halfway through the second box, so I don't run out. Also, your local pharmacy might stock an emergency box for you; mine said they would.

The link that follows is a very good guide to helping an ostomate (someone who has gone through a similar surgical procedure) in returning to a normal lifestyle. I actually looked up similar links and read them to my partner before the surgery. It did take a bit for things to heal up, flexibility being one of the bigger issues. Stretching exercises are helping with that.

> www.ostomyguide.com/a-guide-to-sex-with-an-ostomy/

Some Hiccups

After all this, I did have a couple of hiccups. They didn't get all the cancer, and I had to do six more months of chemotherapy. One of the chemos left me with numb feet and ringing in my ears. I was in the hospital twice, once not being able to swallow, and the next round with a nosebleed that did not want to stop. Because of the chemo drug cisplatin, my platelets had dropped to almost nothing. My doctor took me off of it and switched me to the pill form of the 5-FU (Xeloda). After that, my PET scan showed no cancer, but I had a couple of fatty spots show up on my pancreas and liver. They decided to wait on removing the intravenous port they had put in for some of the chemo treatments.

Two years out from the last of the chemo, I finally had my port removed. I was ecstatic about it. It helped me feel that I was truly recovering from this journey. There were times I wasn't so sure I would make it.

"Butt Support" and Patient Portals

To help me through all this, I set up a personal support page on Facebook. It's called "Butt Support," and it's a closed group (members only). Part of this was so I could keep my family and friends informed on what was going on and not have to keep repeating it. The other part was so I could separate this from my everyday life. Having cancer or any major health issue becomes your life if you aren't careful; being able to have a way to separate from it does help. I saw this with my mother before she passed. The doctors and hospitals were her social life—I didn't want that. I also encouraged my friends to put obnoxious butt jokes on the page. I felt it was important to have a sense of humor about all this. We have to laugh at it, better than crying or feeling sorry for ourselves.

Some of my most "out-there" friends turned out to be some of the people I was in the Army with. They really helped me through this with their weird sense of humor.

Something I found very useful was the patient portals they now have for the hospitals and the Veterans Affairs Program (VA). Yes, I went through the VA for my cancer treatment, even with all the bad press they have received lately. They saved my life, and I was treated well, but I did do my part to keep them on their toes—and I would suggest that be done with any hospital. I used the MyHealtheVet portal the VA offers, as well as the MyChart provided by the Scott and White Hospital. I was able to log in and see my medical record. These are programs that encourage partnering with your healthcare team. You can check over your labs, read doctors' notes, and can have viable questions ready for the doctors when you go to your appointments. I would strongly recommend people who have access to these medical record programs consider them, as they can help you keep on top of your health (and you can double-check the doctors as well!). Most hospitals have a similar program; if they don't say anything about them, ask.

Having Fun With It

There are a few things I like to have fun with. For one, when people ask me about some of what I've been through, I say, "They removed an asshole from my life; unfortunately, it was my favorite one. I was attached to it for over 50 years." Other responses I liked were, as I mentioned above, telling doctors who were examining me that "anal probes are not my fetish," and describing that my anatomy is now a "Frankenstein Barbie Butt." When my hair was falling out, I would tell my friends I was a zombie as I reached up and pulled a chunk of hair out. I left pictures of captured fairies taped behind clear canisters in waiting areas, and I drew pictures of dragons, flaming cancer demons, and one of the aliens doing anal probes. I even told my radiologist after the brachytherapy treatment, "It wasn't right that she drugged me and took advantage of me and never even offered me a movie or dinner."

Two years out now from the last chemo, am I 100%? No. Am I alive and progressing? Yes. I have to watch my hydration; I'm working on getting my strength back, dealing with depression because my recovery is not going fast enough to suit me, and having to face what I may never be able to do again. My boyfriend used to call me his whirlwind. I was proud to be in my late fifties and still keep up with people in their 30s and 40s. Now I have to learn to sit back and watch instead of do. I am planning on being the whirlwind again.

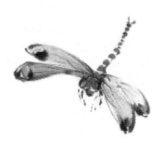

Chapter 9

Pelvic Radiation Disease: The Basics

Angela G. Gentile

Pelvic radiation disease (PRD) is defined by the Pelvic Radiation Disease Association (PRDA) in the UK (*prda.org.uk*) as "any brief or long-lasting problems, which can be anything from very mild to very severe, arising in normal, non-cancerous tissues and which start as a result of radiotherapy to a tumor in the pelvis." The injuries could include bowel or bladder incontinence; diarrhea with urgency or frequency; wind, bloating, abdominal pain, or rectal bleeding; and sexual health difficulties.

"Radiation proctitis" is a primary feature, which is inflammation and damage to the lower parts of the colon. Painful defecation (having a bowel movement) is one of the features of radiation proctitis.

PRD may occur any time following radiotherapy, but sometimes side effects aren't evident for months and even years later. Radiation enteropathy can affect gastrointestinal, genitourinary and sexual functioning. Sometimes it is temporary; other times it is chronic (Wikipedia, retrieved 10 Jul 2018).

Pelvic Radiation Disease is also known as:

- ❖ Pelvic Radiation Injury
- ❖ Pelvic Radiation Damage
- ❖ Late Effects of Pelvic Radiotherapy
- ❖ Side Effects of Pelvic Radiotherapy
- ❖ Radiation Enteropathy
- ❖ Radiation Enteritis

In an article on the PRDA website called "Why does pelvic radiation disease happen?" (2010), it is stated:

"To be certain of killing a tumor, the radiotherapy has to include some of the surrounding healthy tissue. Radiotherapists plan how they will deliver the radiotherapy to each individual very carefully to minimize as far as possible damage to normal tissue but is it an inevitable consequence of radiotherapy that some healthy tissues will be exposed to potentially damaging radiation. Sometimes this causes few problems, at other times it causes damage to critical structures.

Our understanding of how damage to healthy tissue develops has grown. Radiation-induced injury is like a complex wound that will not heal properly. A small number of pioneers around the world have worked to improve our understanding of how this 'complex wound' develops and what steps are effective to try to get it to heal."

Dr. H. J. Andreyev, a gastroenterologist, has done extensive research on the damage done by radiation to the pelvic region. Although necessary to rid the body of cancer, radiation often leaves injury in its wake.

In an article he titled "Gastrointestinal (GI) Consequences of Cancer Treatment: a Clinical Perspective" (2016), Andreyev states that the "medical and research community remains largely uninterested in pelvic radiation disease (PRD), a condition that affects half a million patients every year after radiotherapy for pelvic cancer." He emphasizes the fact that more patients develop PRD than inflammatory bowel disease.

"Curing or controlling cancer without addressing quality of life is no longer acceptable when half of all patients diagnosed with cancer live for ten years after treatment. For those patients afflicted with PRD, it can cause significant misery, and this situation is unacceptable; investment in training and research cannot be delayed any longer." –Dr. H. J. Andreyev

In an article by Morris and Haboubi (2015) called "Pelvic Radiation Therapy: Between Delight and Disaster," the authors identify how the burden of PRD-related symptoms affect a person's quality of life, and how this topic is sub-optimally managed. Their awareness of this important topic also identifies vaginal stenosis as one of the potential radiation-induced injuries. They advocate for "awareness of PRD and the vast potential there is to improve current service provision and research activities."

I've known some cancer specialists in North America who prefer to call the radiation damage done to the gastrointestinal tract "pelvic radiation injury" and recognize and treat individual components. Dr. Foster Lasley, a radiation oncologist, states there are blanket interventions that can help with multiple conditions, such as Trental, Vitamin E, or hyperbaric oxygen therapy, but many of the conditions have individual interventions for treatment. He adds that, unfortunately, some situations do not have any treatment options.

An article in the Lancet describes the problem with not recognizing "radiation-induced toxicity." First, radiation-induced toxicity is not seen as a disease, but as a constellation of vague and poorly defined symptoms. Second, the terminology used to describe and measure these changes after radiation to the pelvic area is often imprecise, leading to misunderstanding, confusion and myth (Andreyev, Wotherspoon, Denham, & Hauer-Jensen 2010).

Carol Anne Hollen, who is living with pelvic radiation disease (PRD), is a USA advocate for PRD using proven protocols from Dr. Andreyev's clinical PRD studies in the UK. She says gastroenterologists (doctors with specialized training in diseases of the gastrointestinal tract and liver) are key to recognizing and treating the disease. The gastrointestinal tract includes the esophagus, stomach, small intestine, colon and rectum, pancreas, gallbladder, bile ducts and liver.

From Hollen's experience, she states top doctors in many cities in the USA recognize and treat PRD. PRD can also be a progressive degenerative disease, which, if diagnosed early, can be adequately treated.

Hollen has learned about a low-FODMAP diet, which is the go-to diet for issues caused by radiation damage. FODMAP stands for

"Fermentable Oligo-, Di-, Mono-saccharides and Polyols," in other words, short-chain carbohydrates that some people cannot digest. Everyday foods like milk, wheat, many fruits and vegetables, legumes and other sugars can cause gas, bloating, diarrhea, constipation, and stomach pain in someone who is intolerant. A low-FODMAP diet can help lessen these symptoms. This diet has mostly been studied in patients with irritable bowel syndrome.

The Pelvic Radiation Disease Association in the UK provides many online resources and documents for both patients and healthcare professionals, including patient handouts on "Exercises for improving bowel control" (which includes sphincter exercises) and "Improving the way your bowel works, for people with constipation" (including instruction on the brace technique, which helps you open your bowel more easily.)

****

REFERENCES:

Andreyev, H. J. (2016). GI Consequences of Cancer Treatment: A Clinical Perspective. *Radiat Res*, 185(4): 341-8. doi: 10.1667/RR14272.1

Andreyev, H. J., Wotherspoon, A., Denham, J. W., and Hauer-Jensen, M. (2010). Defining Pelvic-Radiation Disease for the Survivorship Era. *Lancet Oncol*, 11(4): 310-2. doi: 10.1016/S1470-2045(10)70026-7.

Morris, K. A. L. And Haboubi, N. Y. (2015). Pelvic Radiation Therapy: Between delight and disaster. *World Journal of Gastrointestinal Surgery*, 7(11); 279-288. doi: 10.4240/wjgs.v7.i11.279

Chapter 10

Living With
Pelvic Radiation Disease

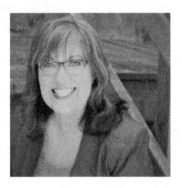

Laura Zick-Mauzy

I wish I could tell you that I am completely and blissfully enjoying my cure. I am not. With that being said, it does not mean I'm ungrateful. Anal cancer has introduced me to so many amazing friends with unparalleled camaraderie. I am thankful for my life, the precious time spent with family, and for the experience. While that may sound strange (and I don't mean I'm happy I got cancer), I'm grateful for what cancer taught me.

However, the late effects of radiation have been physically and emotionally draining. The post-radiation damage to my pelvic region and lymph nodes has left me with physical damage known as Pelvic Radiation Disease (PRD) and psychological scars very much like Post Traumatic Stress Disorder (PTSD). It's called Civilian PTSD, Non-Military PTSD or Non-Combat PTSD.

Pelvic radiation disease (PRD) is not widely recognized in the United States. I believe the reason is that symptoms vary widely, and many patients may not discuss these late side effects with their oncologist or primary care physician. Radiation to the pelvic area also causes damage to neighboring healthy organs and tissues. The damage causes scarring as the body heals. As frustrating as it is, long-term side effects may not present until months, or even years, after radiotherapy completion.

PRD can consist of one or more of these symptoms:

- Bladder dysfunction: urgency and incontinence
- Bowel dysfunction: urgency and incontinence
- Chronic diarrhea
- Hormonal changes
- Early menopause (women)
- Sexual dysfunction
- Vaginal stenosis in women
- Vaginal dryness in women
- Erectile problems in men (blood supply vessels damaged) (Malatek, 2012)
- Infertility/Sterility (Malatek, 2012)
- Decreased libido (Malatek, 2012)
- Lymphedema (poor lymph fluid circulation because of damage to lymph nodes)
- Pelvic bone fragility
- Hairline fractures caused by the radiation
- Brittleness caused by the radiation
- Long-term fatigue (Malatek, 2012)
- Small bowel obstructions (Malatek, 2012)
- Fistulas (an abnormal connection between what should be two hollow spaces) generated by the damage or weakening of the tissue and linings of structures between organs (Malatek, 2012)
- Recurrent urinary tract infections (RARE) (Malatek, 2012)

In my case, the resulting long-term side effects are fatigue, urinary urgency, fecal urgency and incontinence, vaginal stenosis, lymphedema (primarily in my left lower leg), and emotional and social repercussions from those mentioned above. So, here we go: the good, the bad, and the ugly. I will address each of the side effects as they pertain to me and share with you how I handle(d) them.

Fatigue (a.k.a. Tiredness)

I am now five years post-treatment and never regained my precancer energy. I would say I've lost about 30% of my stamina and vitality. This is not the case with all anal cancer survivors, but for me, it seems I'm tired so much of the time—occasionally to the point of falling asleep while driving. Scary stuff.

Here's the thing, though: I sleep well at night. No tossing and turning. There aren't any frequent trips to the bathroom. I don't struggle to fall asleep or to stay asleep. I have dreams. I even had a sleep study and a nocturnal oximetry test (a measure of oxygen saturation), and everything physiologically is in good working order. Extra sleep does not provide any extra energy.

My chronic clinical depression, which I have battled with since my early twenties, is very well controlled with medication, and there hasn't been an onset of recent events to trigger "a newly depressive state" (which might account for increased fatigue). My blood counts are perfect—no anemia (a deficiency in red blood cells). Thyroid, liver and kidney function is normal. I do not have fibromyalgia, chronic fatigue, or Epstein Barr.

I'm pretty much perfect, except for being exhausted. So, what's a girl (or guy) to do? I tried energy drinks, massive doses of caffeine tablets, all kinds of over-the-counter stimulants. Absolutely nothing has worked. I am a lot of things, but lazy is not one of them. Yet, I've portrayed myself as such because of constant fatigue.

Over the course of about a year, my primary care physician has listened to me, empathized with me, and worked alongside me to try to resolve this. Although I have accepted the fact I will never be my former energetic self, there has finally been some progress. He prescribed a medication that stimulates the central nervous system to help me feel more alert and awake. Some days it seems to be more effective than others, but I haven't fallen asleep while driving since taking it. Thank you, doc!! I've also reduced my sugar consumption and made strides in eating healthier. Whenever humanly possible, I push myself (translated: FORCE myself) to move—to do something active—whether it is taking a short walk, painting, or cleaning out a closet—I'm trying to move more. Since energy can neither be created nor destroyed, it's dormant in me somewhere, right? I simply needed to change it from one form (stored) to another (actuated). That's not science; that's just my own crazy explanation . . . ha ha.

Urinary Frequency and Urgency (a.k.a. I Have to Go NOW!)

I have to pee. I have to pee a lot. I know where nearly every restroom is in every store at the shopping mall. And, in the event I'm traveling, and I'm unfamiliar with my surroundings, guess what?! There's actually an app for that! I'm serious! It's called "Toilet Finder." What a wonderful discovery, that app. It's designed for

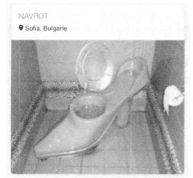

users to add where public toilets are located. There are over 130,000 facilities currently listed, and some users have even posted photos of "unusual" bathrooms from around the world. Pictured here is a photo of one in Sofia, Bulgaria. User Navrot submitted it, and the toilet is in the shape of a lady's shoe. Not really sure if I could pee in there!

I don't have absolute urinary incontinence. In other words, I don't spontaneously lose bladder control without warning. It is difficult, if not impossible, to hold it for an extended period, but there is a warning. My muscle tone is unable to do what it is intended to do. In this case, Kegel exercises (for the pelvic floor) are the first line of defense.

To do Kegel exercises (Cherney, 2013):

1. Try stopping your urine mid-stream when going. The muscles you use are pelvic floor muscles. This is what you'll focus on contracting during Kegel exercises.

2. Focus on tightening those muscles when you have an empty bladder. Hold this position for about five seconds at a time. Relax the muscles and then repeat five times. As your muscles get stronger, increase the duration to 10 seconds of 10 repetitions. Perform the exercises 10 or more times a day.

3. Breathe normally when doing these exercises.

4. Avoid squeezing your stomach, thighs, or buttocks instead of your pelvic floor muscles.

Fecal Urgency and Incontinence (a.k.a. Poop Accidents)

My first experience with bowel incontinence was in a public place. It was absolutely horrible. Picture this . . . My husband and I are out of town with a realtor, looking at a nice house for possible purchase. Uh oh! I felt the undeniable urgency. Immediate panic flooded my soul. But alas! I could just use the homeowner's bathroom, right? WRONG. The water had been turned off at this house!!!

With a look of complete terror on my face, I grabbed my husband and screamed as quietly as I could, "We have to go NOW!" Before we made it to our vehicle, I had an accident.

We quickly drove to a nearby fast food restaurant so I could bolt myself in the bathroom to get reasonably cleaned up. As my luck would have it, the ladies room was occupied, so my husband acted as a guardsman and I went into the men's room for about 20 minutes. Before I came out, I had washed out my pants as best as I could, dried them with the hand air dryer, cleaned the floor and toilet seat . . . TWICE . . . then buried my underwear in the bottom of the waste can . . . they were beyond saving. When I finally emerged from the restaurant, with red eyes and damp pants, I saw that the realtor followed us there! I'm sure the realtor knew what had happened, although he did not know WHY it happened.

I truly wanted to die. Right there. Just kill me. I cried hysterically again. My husband tried desperately to console me, but I was angry. Very angry! Was this how it would be from now on? I asked my husband to get rid of the realtor (I couldn't face him, and I wasn't sure I was "done").

We did not make an offer on the house. To be truthful, we really weren't in there long enough to give it a fair inspection, and there was no way I would face that dear man again. I could not bear to look him in the eyes. Although we did look at a couple other houses later in the year, nothing panned out for us. We eventually bought an affordable commercial building for my photography studio and, oddly enough, we made a home upstairs. What started out as a light-hearted "what if," came to fruition, and we couldn't be happier with our home.

Managing Incontinence

After another public episode a couple months later, I resigned to the fact that, for the time being, I would have to purchase and wear pull-ups. I had to. I just had to.

Disposable underwear.

Depends®.

Diapers.

Whatever you want to call them. I call them beyond lifeworthy embarrassing.

After the emotional trauma of all that, I began researching. I had no clue as to the number of people going through that exact same thing. That both shocked and saddened me.

IT NEEDS TO BE TALKED ABOUT. In fact, this is being written because of the prompting and encouragement of a reader and fellow anal cancer warrior. Others see us as we are on the outside on a day-to-day basis. Women all prettied up with their makeup, hair perfectly coiffed and well-dressed as we go about our business. Men may be clean-shaven and donning their suits as they head to the workplace daily. After all, we don't have cancer anymore. This is the perception the public has of us. We are over it. Cancer is in the past. We are fine now.

NO.

WE ARE NOT.

First, please understand that you are not alone. I am learning that nearly everyone who has had pelvic radiation experiences some degree of incontinence. So, whether or not people are sharing this fact, it is occurring.

Secondly, and think about this, stores like Walmart, Target, Walgreens, etc. carry incontinence products for a reason . . . because they are needed. If there were no demand for them, the retail market would not carry them.

When I first began entertaining the thought of incontinence products, this is what I had envisioned—a large, bulky diaper with Velcro® tabs that made a swish-swish noise when I walked. The thought of pulling those up around my hips was depressing and traumatizing.

Below are some options that I found to be more appealing:

For Women

- Silhouette® (by Depend®)—they are pull-ups that are fitted and made from a cloth-like fabric
- Washable & reusable lace-trimmed incontinence panty (by Wearever®). They come in black, beige, or white, and are for light to moderate incontinence
- Boutique Incontinence pants (by Always® Discreet)—they are actually pretty and have an odor lock protection
- Fannypants® Ladies Freedom Incontinence Bikini Briefs— washable up to 200 times but only hold about three ounces, so these are definitely more for urinary leaks

For Men

- Real Fit® (by Depend®)—they have a finished waistband and a cotton-like fabric
- Protective men's briefs (by TENA®)—these have vertical stripes and are snug-fitting
- Classic Briefs (by Wearever®)—washable and reusable, these have an elastic waistband
- Fannypants® Men's Orca Incontinence Briefs—washable up to 200 times but only hold about three ounces, so these are definitely more for urinary leaks

After the initial shock, the peace of mind that came was worth it. And I would imagine this is better than having a colostomy bag. So . . . I took a deep breath, pulled up my big girl panties, and went on with life . . .

I thought that would be my new normal, but it wasn't. I stumbled upon a medication formulated to lower cholesterol and reduce bile salts. It is sometimes given to people with Irritable Bowel Syndrome with Diarrhea (IBS-D), Dumping Syndrome, and after gallbladder removal. I wondered if it might help me. I discussed the possibility with my physician, and he agreed it was worth trying. This medication is called Questran (cholestyramine). It has been a game-changer for me. Although I still have chronic urgency, I have little diarrhea now. Hallelujah!!! That has helped me to become more confident, and I am beginning to feel a bit "safer" when taking short trips and while working.

Lymphedema

When pelvic radiation damages nearby lymph nodes, or when it is necessary to have nodes removed because of cancer, the result can be a disruption in the flow of protein-rich lymph fluid. The lymphatic system is part of both the immune system and the circulatory system. Lymph fluid contains a type of infection-fighting white blood cells called lymphocytes, and it circulates in the lymphatic vessels instead of the blood vessels.

There are hundreds of lymph nodes throughout our body. When the lymph fluid reaches a node, the nodes work like little filtration centers and filter out any foreign cells or bacteria that may be causing infection. The filtered lymph fluid then returns to circulation throughout the body.

When the body does not filter and circulate the fluid as it was designed, swelling from fluid retention (edema) may occur. When there is swelling, there is less oxygen. Your tissues need oxygen to heal. If, for example, the pelvic nodes have been damaged, lymphedema may present in the legs or feet after the completion of radiation treatments.

It was about three months after treatment when this developed in my lower legs. The left leg is worse than my right. It is unattractive and uncomfortable. I am told that the incidence of lymphedema caused by radiation is equal to the incidence caused by surgical removal of nodes. Other symptoms of lymphedema include pitting (when the skin is pressed, an indentation remains), skin discoloration, pain from swelling, and skin breakdown (an increased risk when wearing compression garments). Unfortunately, there is no "cure" for it, but there is treatment!

I have learned I need to wear compression stockings. There are different types, brands, compressions, lengths, styles, and colors. I was measured by a lymphedema specialist to know what I needed to get. She took measurements of the circumference of my ankle, my calf just below the knee, and my thigh. From there, it was determined I should wear a MEDIUM. Based on the degree of lymph fluid I was retaining, I needed a compression of 20-30 mmHg (20-30 millimeters of pressure of mercury is a pressure reading of blood pressure—like when a nurse is pumping up a blood pressure cuff and watching the needle on the gauge—he/she is watching the mmHg pressure rise).

I wear beige thigh high stockings and prefer the open toe. Since I love my sandals, this allows me a lot more freedom to wear them. My favorite brand is Juzo®. I need to wear them every day. Every. Single. Day. With dresses. With shorts. With leggings, jeans, everything. I was intimidated at first when people gave me "that look" of inquisitiveness. Now, it doesn't bother me because I do

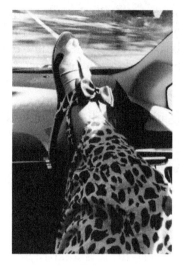

what I need to do. I am who I am—and I have overcome a lot, and that's really something I can take pride in. Compression stockings and all. The compression does not "fix" the problem; it simply helps manage the fluid. One little helpful hint I have learned to help get them on (for open toe people): get a piece of satin or silk and wrap that around your foot before attempting to put the stocking on. It will go on the foot SO MUCH EASIER! Then, grab the fabric at the toe after your stocking is in place and pull it out . . . voila!

I have learned while traveling I must take a break about every two hours to walk around. This is to prevent the risk of developing a blood clot.

I have learned wounds do not easily heal. I fell and had a cut on my shin. At the time of this writing, it has been five weeks, and the wound is still not closed. While I was changing my bandage one day, a slightly blood-tinged watery fluid ran all the way down my leg. That was lymph fluid.

I have learned I must take very good care of my skin. It should be hydrated with a gentle, hypoallergenic lotion. I say that because if there were any sensitivity to a lotion or cream, an allergic reaction would impose potentially serious skin problems. Also, petroleum-based products can break down compression garments, and they are too expensive to replace unnecessarily too soon.

I have learned a massage technique called manual lymph drainage is beneficial in moving lymph fluid. This is not a deep tissue massage. It is a gentle technique performed by someone trained in doing so.

I have learned I may be prone to cellulitis and bacterial or fungal infections. My lymph specialist even recommends I not go barefoot on the beach. If I do remove my compression stockings while on the beach, I do so for only a short period. Now that was hard to hear because I adore the beach, and the sand is an integral part of the experience.

Vaginal Stenosis

Not only is my rear end messed up, but so is my front end (I sound like a poorly designed vehicle, right?). The radiation damage caused scarring to my vaginal canal. I was not aware this would happen, and I found out when my husband and I had sex for the first time after treatments ended. It was EXCRUCIATING. I cried. I tried. It was too much to bear. I would never have sex again. I supposed I would have to hire a mistress for my husband. Yes, I was irrational. I was hurting, embarrassed, and in shock.

MONTHS LATER, I was willing to try again with the game plan of well-lubricating. We slathered and greased and slicked until Vesuvius was surely ready to be mounted. Wrong. It made no difference. My vaginal canal was just too narrow and beat-up to allow it. I was extremely discouraged and disheartened. Again, more tears.

My husband, being the amazing man he is, encouraged me and assured me if we could never have sex again, it would be okay. He understood. He saw the pain was real, and his heart broke for me. That's not what I wanted, though. And I was pretty sure that—given the option—he wouldn't choose it either.

So, my husband got on the Internet and began researching. Much to my surprise, he learned quite a bit. He is the one who told me about vaginal stenosis, and he is the one who told me about vaginal dilators. As I have since talked with women from around the country, many oncologists or radiology oncologists speak to their patients about this and educate them, even recommending that women invest in a set of these dilators.

Vaginal Dilators: What are they? And how do they work?

Vaginal dilators are medical grade, hypoallergenic plastic or silicone tube-shaped vaginal inserts that come in a set of increasing sizes. The small one is very narrow, about the size of a tampon. This is the starting point. You lubricate the dilator and gently insert it into the vaginal canal. I found it most comfortable while lying down and trying to relax. When the dilator has been inserted, contract your muscles to hold it in there. Keep it inside for 5-10 minutes and then remove. Wash with mild soap and warm water. Repeat this process three or four times a week. When the smallest one becomes "too" comfortable, go up to the next size.

More information can be found on the Internet by searching Memorial Sloan Kettering Cancer Center, "How to Use a Vaginal Dilator." I purchased my set online at *vaginismus.com/* for $44.95 (price subject to change.)

Although it took quite a while to get to where I needed to be, I have to say, these were a life saver. All is well. <<wink wink>>

Where I Am Today

In 58 days from this writing, provided God continues bestowing His mercy on me, I will have had my "last" PET/CT scan that will give me the 5-year NED (no evidence of disease) status. My oncologist will say I am cured. I will never use those words, but the 5-year mark is an important one nonetheless.

I continue to paint, write, and do photography. In a few years, I hope to retire from my career as a medical laboratory scientist. Life is good overall. I have a strong faith and support system of family and friends around me. I wish all readers a healthy life and remember, you are not alone. It is a tough journey . . . but it is doable.

"Don't be afraid; just believe."

–Mark 5:36b NIV

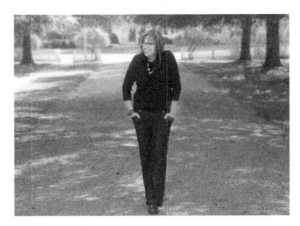

****

REFERENCES:

Andreyev, H.J., Wotherspoon, A, Denham, J. W., Hauer-Jensen, M. (2010). Defining pelvic-radiation disease for the survivorship era. *Lancet Oncol,* 11:310-312 [PubMed]

Malatek, Daniel (2012). "Late Effects of Radiation Therapy Video Transcript." University of Texas MD Anderson Cancer Center. https://www.mdanderson.org/transcripts/poe-radiation-late-effects-malatek.htm

Frazzoni, L; La Marca, M.; Guido, A.; Morganti, A.G.; Bazzoli, F. and Fuccio, L. (2015). Pelvic Radiation Disease: Updates on Treatment Options. *World Journal of Clinical Oncology,* Dec. 10; 6(6): 272-280.

Cherney, Kristeen (13 Sep 2013). "What Home Remedies Work for an Overactive Bladder?" HealthLine. https://www.healthline.com/health/overactive-bladder/home-remedies

Morris, K. A. L. and Haboubi, N. Y. (27 Nov 2015). Pelvic Radiation Therapy: Between Delight and Disaster. *World Journal of Gastrointestinal Surgery,* 11(7).

Zick-Mauzy, Laura (16 Apr 2015). "Pullin' Up My Big Girl Panties,"
Anal About Cancer (blog).
https://analaboutcancer.com/pullin-up-my-big-girl-panties/

RESOURCES:

Memorial Sloan Kettering Cancer Center. "How to Use a
Vaginal Dilator." https://www.mskcc.org/cancer-care/patient-
education/how-use-vaginal-dilator

Pelvic Radiation Disease Association in the UK
(*prda.org.uk*)

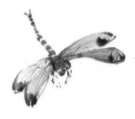

Chapter 11

How My Story Helped and Inspired Others

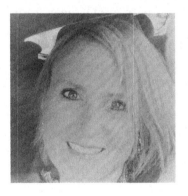

Jodi Canaday Green, Ed. D.

On October 22, 2013, I entered the ever-growing community of people diagnosed with cancer. In the middle of an impersonal doctor's office, where I waited 45 minutes past my appointment time, I had to hear the words, "you have anal cancer." All I could think of when I was sitting in that small room was "Please get me out of here." Cancer was not common in my family, and for me to hear those words at 38 years old was terrifying. I had two small tumors, and I was diagnosed with stage 1 squamous cell carcinoma.

First I Cried and Prayed

The first thing I did, besides cry, was pray. I prayed for peace, guidance, doctors, anything I could think of to pray about. Following that first prayer, I went straight to my job. At the time I was a middle school assistant principal. I had been going to doctor appointments secretly. The principal and secretary knew I was having issues and the extent, but no one else knew I was having all these butt procedures (not something you talk about in a faculty meeting).

I pulled my staff together and told them I had been to the doctor and was just diagnosed with anal cancer. I told them I didn't know the details, didn't know the treatment, and didn't know what was going to happen. I told them I would become a Relay For Life advocate and wear the ribbon proudly, even though I didn't know the color (which my principal suggested was brown . . . LOL).

The quiet that covered the room was scary. At that time, one of the teachers asked to pray for me. Most of the 50 faculty and staff members gathered around in a circle in the middle of the school library, while touching myself or my husband, and began praying for healing.

So Many Doctors

Did you know when you have cancer you have so many doctors that it's hard to know what all they do? I had no idea. I was very lucky to know a teacher whose wife worked for a cancer center in the heart of Nashville was able to fast-track me to some of the best of the best.

The first doctor I got in to see was the oncology surgeon. This doctor is the one who does your surgeries. Well, my doctor was Richard Geer. Yes, Richard Geer. He may not look like the actor Richard Gere you know about, but he was a very nice-looking gentleman. I went to his office first for an examination to determine the extent of my tumors. After the examination, we began talking about other treatment. Just a few days later, Dr. Geer placed my port so I could start treatment.

The medical oncologist, Dr. Dianna Shipley, was from my home state of West Virginia. Imagine the connection we had—being in a big city far away with a common place to call home. She placed a chemo pump on my left side, into my port, that remained there until the conclusion of treatment.

Last was my radiation oncologist. Dr. Nguyen prepared me for 35 radiation treatments that changed my life forever. Never in my wildest dreams did I realize the damage radiation could do to a body. Not only were those damages physical, but the aftereffects also hurt my emotional well-being. Where I could go and what I could do was limited due to those radiation treatments.

Support from Friends and Family

I have four children, and at the time of diagnosis, their ages ranged from 5-18. Hunter, the oldest, was 18. A senior in high school with a life of his own, he made a point of checking on me daily to ask how I was. Alexi, 16, a high school sophomore, played varsity soccer and had her entire team purchase shirts to support my fight and me. Emma Claire, my youngest daughter, was 8 and in third grade. The word cancer was so scary to an 8-year-old, but her teacher was amazing at making sure she felt safe and loved and that she understood I was going to be okay. The youngest, Jonas, was 5 and full of life. He just wanted Mommy to feel better. My husband continued to work and appreciated all the people who stepped up to help.

When I knew I was going to have to take a leave of absence from work, each department of my faculty adopted one of my children and showered them with gift cards, coloring books, and toys. They did the things for them that I was not capable of doing.

As I was still processing this whole thing, I had many people reach out to me. Many asked what they could do to help me through this process. Some very special people in my life stopped what they were doing to become my caregivers. My mother took a leave of absence from her job three states away to help my family. My college best friend came to my house for a week and made sure my children had a Thanksgiving. My husband's cousin drove 500 miles to spend three days taking me to treatments. My sister, my sweet sister, made a radiation countdown. In this countdown was a letter full of childhood memories that was opened every day to make me smile before every treatment. A dear friend set up a meal train so my family would be taken care of nightly throughout the week. My faculty cooked Thanksgiving dinner and had it waiting to be picked up in my office. A custodian who worked at my school, a childhood friend, and all of those mentioned above transported me daily to radiation treatments and took over as a role model for my four children.

I was so blessed to have so many friends and family by my side to help in any way that I needed. The only thing I asked of them early on was to set a reminder to pray for my family because once the newness of my diagnosis wore off, they would all go on about their lives while my family would still be fighting for a new normal. They did not disappoint.

My Story Helped and Inspired Hundreds of Others

Social media became my outlet, and this is where I learned my story was touching the lives of others. I remember one of my first posts:

"On our way to my treatment this afternoon, we stopped by the school, and my staff were wearing matching 'Go Green' shirts with our Mustang logo. It was so moving for me to see them all together. A pep rally was scheduled for the end of the day. I walked into the gym to see all the staff matching, and they all came together to have their picture taken with me . . . I am sooo blessed to have a staff and faculty who come together when things happen. We (Mr. Powell and myself) explained to the student body my diagnosis (cancer) and told them I would be back in January. It was such a moving moment. I love those kids, and I love my staff." *CaringBridge*

Journal Entry

That was the first moment I realized my diagnosis could do more than affect my health. It was bringing together hundreds of children and adults.

I updated a CaringBridge site weekly. One week, about a month into treatment, I received a message from a young man I had grown up with whom I had not spoken to in years about how he had been struggling with weight loss. His message read,

"I have been dealing with a few things in my life that, without a doubt, pale in comparison to what you and your family have been going through. With that being said, I wanted to say thank you! Your attitude is so uplifting and inspiring, it gives me a tremendous amount of strength to do what I need to do. You are amazing and provide a wonderful example to us all. You prove that we all have choices in how we live each day, and the example you set truly touches my heart."

He kept up with my Facebook posts and CaringBridge and later told me he knew if I could have such a calm spirit and positive outlook while fighting cancer, he could work harder to reach his goals. Wow. I had no idea I was making that big of a difference in the lives of others.

Many times, after treatment I would run in to people I knew, and that is a lot of people working in the public school system for 15+ years. They would always mention how I had motivated them to get a check-up, reminded them life is short and to enjoy every moment, or even just stop and play with their children. I had no idea how the impact a cancer diagnosis on myself could affect so many people.

Following every casual encounter I had with someone, the fear I held inside of me faded away little by little. The first day after diagnosis I would repeat the scripture, Psalms 56:3 over and over. In this scripture, it says, "When I am afraid I will put my trust in you." I think I had to be reminded hourly that I needed to put my trust in Christ, but as I heard story after story of how my journey was changing the lives of others, the fear became more bearable.

My Encounters with the Lord Brought Me Peace

Peace overcame me that day I sat in church praying when the Lord spoke to me. In my heart and ear, I heard this small whisper. I don't know what song they were singing or what anyone was saying. It felt as if Jesus himself was sitting behind me in the pew. I audibly heard these words, "I know about suffering . . . I know what good can come from hurt and despair. You have no idea what I am about to do with you. I HATE that you are going to have to go through this, but I am right beside you. I will wipe your tears, kiss your head, and hold you close... But we are going to get through it together. Just hold on . . . hold on . . . what is to come is beyond your comprehension . . . I can't wait . . ." That was when I knew I was in the presence of the Lord. I couldn't wait to tell the world. I posted the experience on social media and told my family.

I also remember sitting on that radiation table during a treatment, tears streaming down my face as I struggled to lie still from the burns the other treatments had caused. The pillow on which I was lying pushed down as if someone was lying right beside me. The chills came over my body, as I knew the Holy Spirit was beside me every step. "Peace, peace, wonderful peace . . ." That hymn resonated in my heart and soul. I posted on social media shortly after this experience the following words,

"I already stand in awe at our God's healing power. His comfort is beyond describable. I have leaned on Psalms 56:3 throughout this journey because fear has consumed me. That all turned to a calmness one day when I was in my radiation treatment. I lay completely still holding a foam ring so that I don't move my arms and hands. My head sits softly on a pillow. About the 10th radiation beam, out of 18, I felt someone lay their head beside my head on that pillow. At that moment my tears flowed because I knew I was in His presence. What a spiritual moment that I was blessed to have."

After feeling a fear that was unexplainable, it was so welcoming to feel a peace that only the Lord Most High could provide. I had never experienced the Lord in such a physical way.

My Life Became "Unnormal"

January 21, 2014, was the day I returned to the doctor to be told he did not see any evidence of disease in my tumor location. Of course, scans and other tests had to be done to get an official report the cancer had been taken care of, but this day is the day that everything in my "normal" life became "unnormal."

I had no idea of the life changes that had taken place during this journey and was so surprised to hear I was in menopause at 38. I didn't realize the intimacy with my husband would be altered. I had no idea going to the bathroom would be as frequent or as urgent as it was and even is still to this day.

I believe people are completely unaware of all cancer does to people. Quality of life following cancer treatment is drastically different, yet people feel since we don't have cancer anymore we are fine, but that is not the case. However, I would rather deal with all the side effects than the alternative. Anal cancer is not kind. It does not hold back. It is life-changing.

Anal Cancer Did Not Beat Me

Not meaning to sound boastful, but I was in my final year of a doctoral program in 2013. I had completed all the course work and was working on my dissertation when I was diagnosed. I had worked far too hard and far too long to let the diagnosis of cancer take that away from me. During treatments, I chose to not focus on the final step, but as soon as the final treatment ended, I was more determined than ever. On April 4, 2014, I successfully defended my dissertation and heard the words, "Congratulations Dr. Green." I will never forget the emotions that escaped my heart the moment I realized I had accomplished something most people don't even attempt. At that very moment, I was the winner!

Our Stories Affect Others

My story is one of many, and my story is one of a kind. How is that? We all have a story to tell. We all have affected one person or many when we are going through our hardest times. We can choose to mope, cry, scream, hate, and complain, or we can decide to pray, worship, stay strong, look for goodness, and find peace. I know when I was supposed to be the most frustrated and angered, I was the calmest. That process not only changed my life but the lives of many others. We all go through storms, and we all make choices on how we are going to handle them.

✳✳✳✳✳✳✳✳✳

REFERENCE:

Join Jodi's Journey–CaringBridge
(caringbridge.org/visit/joinjodisjourney)

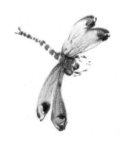

Chapter 12

The Seven Stages of the Cancer Journey

Angela G. Gentile

To me, the word "journey" sounds positive. It's an act of traveling from one place to another. When I think of a trip somewhere, I think of it as an adventurous journey to be enjoyed. Of course, there are bound to be some twists and turns, but what kind of journey is it if it all goes as planned? We often come up against detours, and sometimes it gets scary, especially when we are in unfamiliar territory.

When I was diagnosed with anal cancer in May of 2017, many people, including my radiation oncologist, said I was now on a "journey." On the other hand, I found a lot of violent and war-related terms used when it came to cancer. People diagnosed with cancer are expected to "fight the fight" and become "warriors." We are told cancer can be "beaten." There are many other violent and combative words used for the cancer "battle." How about "slash/poison/burn" to refer to the life-saving treatments of surgery/chemotherapy/radiation therapy. I feel this language does not necessarily help those with cancer and their families; in fact, it can perpetuate fear and anxiety. I am not the combative type, so when faced with this battle, I didn't feel quite prepared.

War Journey

People who are told they have cancer are caught in a strange world of a "war journey." This is such an oxymoron. We are bombarded with contradictory concepts as we grapple with what's happening to us. No wonder those who have cancer struggle with their feelings. No wonder family members, professionals, and other supporters are confused on how to help and support. Being at a loss for words comes naturally.

So, when we are facing a journey of fighting cancer, we have what appears to be a very violent and unpredictable ordeal facing us. It comes with uncertainty. We must call war on cancer and march forward on this emotionally and physically challenging nightmare. Our loved ones encourage us to remain strong and positive on top of it all!

I experienced this cancer nightmare. It was no journey, I tell you. It was hell on earth. The radiation therapy to my pelvic region and systemic chemotherapy to eradicate an anal tumor were brutal. I eventually ended up in the hospital. Thankfully, I was able to complete my treatment regime, but it wasn't pleasant. Fortunately for me, six months post-treatment, I was declared cancer-free.

The emotional upheaval was too much to take sometimes. I faced experiences, thoughts, and feelings I had not yet encountered in my 51 years. The emotional and spiritual impact was way more than I imagined (never mind the physical beating on top of it all!).

Seven Stages

Looking back, I recognize there were phases and turning points in my cancer encounter. There are many medical care transitions that not only affect our physical health but our emotional and spiritual well-being. This so-called "war journey" I was on had me going to deep caverns—dark, scary, cold, and barren places in my soul. Sadness, fear, shame, guilt, numbness, gratefulness, compassion, thankfulness, humility, etc. were all experienced in a matter of months.

There were different phases in my war journey with anal cancer. Some steps in this ordeal were done on my own or with loved ones, while others were done with the help and support of a team.

As I reflect on it, I divide my whirlwind cancer ordeal into seven phases:

1. Getting a Diagnosis (Discovery/Treatment Plan)
2. Awaiting Treatment
3. Treatment Phase
4. Post-treatment (Healing/Recovery)
5. Rehabilitation
6. Getting Good News
7. Back to Life After Cancer (New Normal/Late Effects)

In each of these phases, there are different challenges to overcome and deal with. Some of the segments overlap, and some take longer than others. Each step represents a turning point in the journey. For those embarking on this task, transitioning between each phase can be quick, or it can drag on. Changing gears from one phase to the next can be easy (letting go of the past), or it can be challenging. Each person's journey will be different, and it may or may not include all of these components.

1. Getting a Diagnosis

The first leg of the journey will most likely be shocking. Finding out you have anal cancer causes a lot of fear, anxiety, sadness, and other feelings. Before you get to the diagnosis, there are often symptoms you have been dealing with and tests you have to undergo. This is what I call the discovery phase. It's like an explorer trying to find the answer to something. Soon after the shock of diagnosis comes the requirement to make treatment decisions. This whole process usually happens quickly, as people often don't want to delay, therefore allowing cancer to grow and spread. Then you will decide who to tell, how to tell them, and when to tell them. This will most likely cause some emotional difficulty for you and them.

2. Awaiting Treatment

The second and perhaps one of the most difficult times emotionally for many is the time waiting for the cancer treatment to start. For some people, a few days can feel like forever. It can never come too soon. Delays, schedule conflicts, etc. can also happen, which makes it even more nerve-wracking. It helps to learn how to be in the moment. Meditation or activities that help you focus on other things will help your mental state. There is nothing more harrowing than knowing you have cancer, and there is nothing you can do about it until treatment starts. It can be a frightening time, and your thoughts can get away on you. It may even be hard to sleep or eat.

3. Treatment

Treatment is the busiest time. There will be all kinds of appointments—chemotherapy, radiation therapy, and surgery for some. Managing side effects, pain, and other issues can keep you hopping. You may need to see a "Pain Management Specialist." This is when your feet hit the pavement. Trips to the store to pick up this or that, trying out a new cream or ointment, managing the fatigue, dealing with hair loss issues. There is so much going on during this active medical treatment phase. Go with the flow and take one day at a time. You never know what each day has in store for you. At the end of treatment, there may be a celebration to mark the ending, such as ringing a bell or applause.

4. Post Treatment (Healing/Recovery)

The transition from active treatment to after treatment is the most dramatic turning point. Up until this time you have been very active, busy, task-oriented. Now the appointments are fewer and farther between. You have time now to sit back and say, "Whew! What a ride." The body has to heal from any surgery, chemo, or radiation therapy. This can take six weeks to a year, depending on your body and what was done to it. Some people feel depressed. Others deal with crippling anxiety. An empty or depleted feeling may come on strong, which is discomforting. Numbness, post-trauma fallout, and other heavy feelings may consume you. Waiting to see if the treatment worked may also play on your mind.

5. Rehabilitation

When you start to feel a bit stronger and your appetite improves, you may start feeling like getting more active and back into the real world. Your family and friends will support and encourage your recovery efforts. Getting out of the house, going to the gym, or joining a yoga class may help you feel better. A slow and gradual return to a schedule and active lifestyle can help you start to feel more like yourself again. This recovery happens in baby steps for some people. Your mental health may begin to improve as you start seeing more people and doing some of the things you used to enjoy.

6. Waiting for the News

The follow-up post-treatment tests/scans/exams may consist of a few appointments. The specialist will have some procedures to perform and information to gather to formulate a conclusion if the treatment was successful or not. When those test results come back, and the news is good, this is potentially a highlight and turning point in your cancer journey. You and others may want to celebrate. Some people will have trouble believing it to be true. Others will live in fear of recurrence. (For those who do not receive good news, it's back to the specialists to determine next steps, repeating the first step and determining treatment.)

7. Back to Life After Cancer (New Normal/Late Effects)

After you feel recovered and rehabilitated to a point where you can start getting back to your normal routines (e.g., work, other tasks), you will be reintroduced to previous routines and responsibilities. You may still be dealing with rehabilitation as well. The emotional response to the final portion of this journey, getting back to life after cancer, will vary for everyone. Some people will want to put the cancer experience behind them and move forward without looking back. Others will want to incorporate their newfound knowledge and experiences into their new life and perhaps help others through their journeys. This experience transforms some. Some will be traumatized and worry about recurrence, dealing with feelings of anxiety and fear. Finding a new normal doesn't happen overnight. There will also be possible late effects of treatments that cause some problems physically.

Dealing With Difficulties

We can run into some difficulty if the issues from each phase are not resolved and pile up on each other. There tends to be more distress when the transition happens unsupported. For example, after treatment ends, you may no longer have the daily visits with the radiation team, and the lack of support may have you feeling cut-off and very much alone. The lack of structured medical appointments may have you feeling lost and without a purpose. Sometimes there is no time to process what we are feeling or dealing with. Things can happen quite quickly. The unexpected transitions can cause psychological trauma, so understanding the process can help you cope with it. Paying attention to your thoughts and feelings during each phase can help you determine if you need more support, possibly professional help from a counselor or social worker.

When we are dealing with a medical crisis, we either get better or worse. Sometimes we remain where we are. Time is usually on our side when we seek active treatment and give ourselves time to heal and recover.

When Cancer Returns

For some of us, cancer will recur. This will be the second phase of our cancer journey. We may be able to overcome it; however, some will end up with cancer as a chronic disease, one which is managed over an extended period. For others, cancer will become life-threatening, and we will have to deal with issues regarding the end-of-life transition. Supports are so important at any stage of our cancer experience.

Finding Something Positive

At some point, many of us may decide to look at the positives in our cancer encounter. Reframing what we are going through can help us cope. For me, I wanted to know what I could learn from this. The importance of love, compassion, and connectedness were some of the important lessons I learned. I am forever changed.

The cancer journey is different for everyone, but there are steps we can all relate to. Our emotional responses to each segment of the journey depend on our resilience and strength. We all walk a similar path, but at our own pace. For some, the transitions between phases are more challenging than others. Consider seeking emotional support from others during those challenging times. If you reach out you will never be alone in the cancer experience.

Chapter 13

A Journey Through Darkness

Joy Anderson

For over two years I have traveled in the shadow of death.
Every day now, I poison myself willingly.
My body had been mutilated and changed.
I am the hanged man, unable to do anything but wait.
Soon the waiting will be done.
I will find the strength to cut myself free.
I am not the same anymore.
I have and do face death each day.
No one can come through this without being changed.
I will be stronger, maybe not in body, but in will.
I am not bitter, but have a better understanding of what being alive can mean.
I travel now through the halls of the underworld.
Death is my companion and my friend.
I ask for what was a part of me to die, so that I may live.
As I travel upwards, back to the light, I have time to reflect on things I had thought were important.
I think of friends who have not been true friends.
Family that had not been family.
I know the ones who have reached for me.
Ones who keep pulling me back to the light.

I cry for those I had loved, but who have shown how shallow their love is.

I am blessed by those that have come forward and given me strength, in deeds and words.

The road I am traveling is dark; they have been my light, guiding me back.

As fall approaches, I see the darkness that comes as well.

The darkest time is yet to come.

I am not ready to stay in the underworld.

Come winter will be my rebirth into this world.

By spring I will be seeing the promise of my new life.

I will be very much alive and ready to continue this journey of life.

It would be easy to stay here, to go deeper into the dark.

I give thanks to those that have and are lighting my way back.

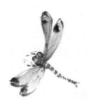

Chapter 14

Swimming Through Psychosis

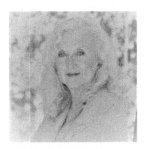

Susan (Sue) Anderson Molenda

H earing bad news can be traumatic. The trauma can have serious effects, which are distressing. You will experience an amazing array of circumstances—life-altering and mind-blowing—whenever or if ever—you are told you have late-stage cancer with a probability of becoming terminal. I did. And I know my response was not typical. But neither was it unique. I had what the psychiatrist called a "brief, reactive psychosis." My mind wasn't able to cope with the news.

The experience was disturbing. I recovered VERY quickly, but I feared I might be marked as "odd, different, weird" forever. I worried I might be stigmatized with the label "mentally ill." And I had cancer. Potentially terminal cancer. That severe diagnosis can make anybody go a little "crazy."

I've been battling rectal (or anal) cancer for eight years as of this writing. Over those eight years, I had a total of three brief psychotic episodes, the latest (and longest) of which happened over three years ago. My adult children were afraid they had lost their mother. Upon viewing videos of myself during the last event, I was appalled. The person living in my body and speaking with my voice was nothing like me.

Over the past several years, I've been writing my book called *Anal Cancer is Really Sh*tty*, available soon on Amazon.com and Audiblebooks.com, in which I dealt lightly with this issue. But as a guest author in this anthology, I will share in greater depth and with equal candor about the horror that accompanies the loss (temporary or otherwise) of certain mental capacities.

I'll discuss the way I fought, each time, to quickly be weaned off of medications and resume a normal life. And I'll reveal how horrifically, in the last of these episodes, my family discovered the stark reality that people perceived as having an irreversible cognitive impairment are violently, or at times, pharmacologically abused by hospital staff, and must be protected from permanent harm or possibly death at the hands of unscrupulous healthcare personnel. Nurses or orderlies who abuse patients physically may expect to get away with the criminal behavior because they think the patients will not have any recollection of the abuse. And then, to your horror, you may find the patient is given a combination of drugs designed to cause permanent memory loss. You may even discover, as my children did, that many of the drugs on the long list of remedies you or your loved one are given have severe warnings about being given at the same time, as the combination may result in severe side effects, including organ damage and even death.

Each episode I experienced had similar coincidences involving certain kinds of anesthesia and pain meds, and every "psychotic" or allegedly "bipolar" event closely followed on the heels of surgical procedures. You or your loved ones may have sensitivities or allergies to certain drugs or drug combinations which can bring on symptoms like depression, anxiety, irritability, hallucinations, and other unusual mental states. Keeping track of similar circumstances accompanying each episode can help you avoid having such complications in the future.

I hope I'm able to share a bit of wisdom, sprinkled freely with humor, hope, and assurance. I hope to inspire you to keep hope very much alive. Hope that you'll survive and beat cancer, and do it with your sanity fully intact. By reading about my experiences and others, I hope you will find relief from much of the anxiety and turmoil by reading our accounts of overcoming various aspects of living with cancer or recovering from it. I have made online and in-person friends of people who joined the same cancer support groups from which I've sought solace. Many people have revealed they find themselves in need of antidepressants or other relief for the types of distress that result from having a diagnosis of a serious, life-altering, and life-threatening condition.

Group members occasionally disclose they too have faced sadness and distress over the new "normal" that overtakes their lives. The possibility of dying from cancer, the viciousness of side effects resulting from cancer treatments, and the financial or relationship challenges they confront are all significant reasons for distress and fear.

In my case, I'd been "proactive" for years. I tried twice to get an early diagnosis, which is reportedly the most significant way of acquiring a potential cure for the disease I feared I was developing. For years, my abdominal pain, rectal pain and bleeding, and grooved stools, coated in streaks of blood, seemed ample evidence to me that something was seriously wrong. I was SURE, for years, I was facing a probable diagnosis of colon or rectal cancer.

I read a book at 37 that convinced me to change my family's diet and lifestyle. We became entirely vegan by ridding the house of every bit of white sugar, white rice, white flour, and white fat. We cut out meat, dairy, and eggs, and bought a Champion Juicer. We sourced enormous bags of carrots and bushels of apples to juice in our quest for clean, cancer-free bowels. We read countless books and watched numerous videos that reinforced our belief that this new, clean diet of mostly organic produce and our avoidance of "junk" food in our diets would protect us against all potential or existing disease or illness. My husband, often pennywise and pound foolish, canceled the family health insurance coverage, believing carrot juice would cure every ill that our children or we might encounter.

I recognized that injuries to our preteen and teenaged kids could easily bankrupt us. It is now "illegal" to go without insurance for our children and ourselves, but back in the 1990s, it was allowed. It was up to the discretion of individuals to decide these things for their own families. As soon as I could afford to, I replaced my husband's employer-offered insurance with my employer's policy. This provided great relief when my daughter developed a serious illness that could not be cured with a glass of carrot juice. My symptoms went away for a couple of years after we changed our diets, but returned, despite consistent avoidance of alleged carcinogenic foods. So I had a colonoscopy at my mother's insistence, at age 39. The doctor said I had "nothing but hemorrhoids and diverticulosis." The rectal pain and bleeding intensified over the years, and I had a second colonoscopy at age 47, but my symptoms were dismissed as "nothing" again.

I divorced my husband at 50 and moved to California. I eventually secured a full-time job with benefits, and I went for another colonoscopy because I was having horrific symptoms, much worse than those at 39 and 47, and I desperately feared the outcome would be worse than I'd previously imagined.

I woke from that third colonoscopy to hear the round-faced gastroenterologist Dr. Fisher say, "I took one look at that mass in your anus, and I said, 'Whoop, she's got anal cancer.' But then we biopsied it, and it was benign, so you're good to go."

I was horrified. I had been dumping gigantic puddles of blood into the toilet at every bowel movement. I'd felt every time I rode a city bus that I was being anally raped with a jackhammer. This could not be "good to go." Not by a long shot.

"What about the pain and the bleeding?" I asked.

Dr. Fisher said, "Well, I'll give you a prescription for some Vicodin, and here's some Analpram. If it's a hemorrhoid, this will shrink the swelling and make you feel better."

"Um . . . Do you . . . biopsy hemorrhoids, usually, Doctor?" I asked.

The very offended doctor harrumphed, "Well, I'll show the films to my associate, and if he feels like there's a reason to call you, he'll call you."

The primary care physician who had referred me to Dr. Fisher exclaimed, "My God, I hope it's not too late! Because you could have, forgive me, CANCER?!!" when I told her my symptoms. That's what I expected to hear. I knew these symptoms were severe indicators of colorectal disease.

I was not in the least upset when I received a call from Dr. Fisher's associate a couple of weeks later saying, "Mrs. Molenda, I'm so sorry to be calling you. I know Dr. Fisher told you your mass was benign, but in my experience with a mass of this size, while there can be a veneer of benign cells on the surface, frequently there is, lurking beneath the surface, a cluster of malignant cells. Those cells can be eating through the muscle wall into the lymph nodes and other tissues below, and from there they can be invading lymph glands and other structures . . . So I'd like to ask you to come back in for a colonoscopy with ultrasound, which will give us a picture of what's going on. I'll take a larger sample for biopsy, and if it's malignant, I'll refer you to an oncologist and surgeon, and get you treated for colorectal cancer."

I was not at all surprised to awaken and have him shove two papers into my hands, saying, "Here are your referrals to your oncologist and surgeon. Call them as soon as possible."

But it WAS a huge shock to find my daughter, later that afternoon, telling me to stop talking with my boyfriend, who apparently had left hours ago, and threatening to call 911 if I didn't stop having this imaginary conversation. I did not know the boyfriend wasn't there.

I did not realize I was losing my grip on reality. I was lying on my bed, trying to imagine what I should say if the police came. When my daughter told me she had called 911, I stood up from my bed, stepped through the screen of the open living room window, and onto the balcony, where I commenced to perform quite an entertaining monologue. (Have I mentioned that I'm an actress? It's the one pursuit I love more than writing.)

I used multiple character voices and accents. My thought was if the police arrived and accused me of "being crazy," I could suddenly curtail the performance and ask, "Am I an actress yet?" Then, I reasoned, surely the police would understand I was just another wannabe actress, coming to Los Angeles in search of an acting career. I thought that would "get me out of the jam" my daughter was creating for me. Because there's nothing crazy about out-acting Robin Williams in an effort to "break in" to the industry to which so many aspire and for which so few qualify to become "stars" on the Hollywood Walk of Fame, from which I lived only blocks away.

Soon, I was in the courtyard of my apartment building, surrounded by a good half-dozen paramedics and law enforcement individuals. I wasn't aware of much at all. Not the least of the things of which I was unaware was the fact that the twilight sleep I'd endured before the procedure was brought on by a drug to which I have significant sensitivity.

I was driven to a nearby hospital with my children following closely behind. I was subjected to multiple CT scans of my brain. They were looking for evidence of traumatic brain injury as an explanation for my sudden loss of sanity. I imagine they found nothing, though I *had* been kicked multiple times by an escaped convict, way back when I was 21. In an exam room, a doctor asked me questions. Not finding anything rational in my responses, the doctor asked the same questions of my adult daughters, and I soon enjoyed another excruciating ride in an ambulance, on my carved-up anus, over bumpy terrain to a mental hospital in Pasadena, where my daughters would visit only occasionally, as it could take hours in L.A. traffic to get there, and where I'd remain for about a week.

It soon became apparent that my faculties had returned, and the psychiatrist released me to go home, but it would be a long while before the insurance company would go ahead and approve my visits with an oncologist and a surgeon. My brother had called the "boyfriend" and urged him to give me "space," which he did by fleeing the country because he had no documents proving he had a right to be on American soil.

Eventually, I was able to see the oncologist, who would tell me my diagnosis of rectal cancer. "I thought it was anal cancer," I said. The "diagnosis" on my referral documents had read, "Malignant neoplasm of the anal canal."

"Same thing," my oncologist shrugged. Eventually, I had a plan for treatment of the disease. I'd have concurrent radiation and chemotherapy, and after healing from the effects of those, there would be surgery to remove the tumor.

I was shocked when the time for surgery came to find I would have to undergo a permanent colostomy. The operation was eventually scheduled, and off I went. I found that after that major surgery, I became emotionally distressed, and a psychiatrist was sent to see me. I was crying and screaming without making much sense. The psychiatrist scribbled, "bipolar" on a form and left the room. I went home from the surgery with a prescription for pain medicine— Vicodin and Percocet. I was in extreme pain and had a hard time keeping track of when and how much pain medicine I was to take.

After a couple of weeks, I found myself again in a distressing condition, emotionally. I was transported to another neighborhood hospital, and I had very little awareness of what was going on. What I was sure of was my son (who had not followed his three sisters and me to live in California) was now parked outside the hospital doors, which I thought were just outside my room and across the hall in a large helicopter, with which he intended to rescue me from my ex-husband, my daughters, and the hospital staff. In my delirium, I was convinced my son was my only ally, and he and I were communicating through a code of musical notes, which I'd sing at the top of my lungs.

Apparently, I was communicating this way on a regular basis, and the nursing staff found it most entertaining. Nurses frequently came in and asked me to sing for them, and I did. I was able to hit higher and louder notes than I'd ever heard issue forth from my lungs. Although the nurses always left laughing, I was very convinced that my son (who was actually not there) must be highly impressed with my newfound operatic skills.

At some point, the antibiotics, which were being used to cure a major abdominal infection, had served their purpose. A doctor came to tell me that my abdomen would be drained of the fluid and pus with the help of a CT-guided needle aspiration procedure. The whole hospital staff assembled to watch, and my returning sanity enabled me to realize they must all be astounded that the operatic lunatic of a few days before had been restored to her right mind. Nobody looked at me funny, and nobody asked me to sing.

I was sent home, and for a while, not another word was said about this second episode of temporary lunacy my daughters had again endured. But I did hear, over the course of a few weeks, that during this episode and the previous occasion, my daughters had feared that I was "gone" forever . . . out of my mind . . . never to return. So they were very adamant I should avoid ever taking those pain-relieving opioids again. When I had another occurrence of cancer a year later, I told the doctors I was allergic to Percocet and Vicodin and could only take Dilaudid for pain, or other drugs in that category.

Several years and many more cancer complications went by before the third and last of my encounters with mental health professionals occurred. I'd had major surgery to remove a large tumor in my buttock and several procedures to try to heal fully from that surgery. I eventually ended up needing a "flap surgery" to try to repair the non-healing wound. The surgeon asked me, "Have you ever had an adverse reaction to anesthesia before?" My answer should have been yes. But, ill-advisedly, I said, "No." I must have been given the wrong kind of anesthesia, and I do not recall going home from that surgery.

I only recall a few days after returning from the hospital, standing next to my middle daughter outside in a rainstorm, screaming "NO!!!" She was screaming back that if I didn't shut up and sleep, she was going to kill herself. I don't recall much of the subsequent conversation with my best friend, who lived across the backyard in the main house. I rent her guesthouse. Apparently, over a few days' time, I'd sunk into an increasing depth of insanity. I don't recall much, but I woke in a mental hospital, wearing a bathrobe I'd just given my best friend for her December 4th birthday and wondering how I came to be wearing it.

I'd apparently crossed the backyard to my friend's back door in the middle of the night, clad only in my top and bra, and with the colostomy bag on my left abdomen and the surgical drain bulb hanging from its rubber hose from my left buttock. I'd gone completely out of my mind.

Police were called. They had taken me, after a lengthy, nonsensical conversation, to the hospital, and my friend, suddenly realizing I was naked from the waist down, had given me her bathrobe to conceal the drain, bag, and hose from the eyes of the distressed cops and paramedics.

This time, my hospital stay was more than a week or two. At an early visit, I'd told the kids a couple of orderlies had beaten me up in the shower. I recall that, vaguely. They shoved me down hard onto the wooden slats of the seat in the shower area, and that had ripped the surgical drain right out of my buttock. I got home weeks later and learned from the post-op instructions on the dining room table, I was not to sit for thirty days. I was to return to the surgeon's office to have my stitches removed fourteen days after the surgery. I'd been in the hospital for thirty days, sitting constantly, and the stitches were not taken out until after that.

Upon returning from the hospital, I was fairly sane, I guess, but remembered very little. I was released from the hospital on Christmas Eve. The hospital sent me home with prescriptions for two medications. My pharmacist told me one of those would negatively interact with my antinausea meds for chemo, so I told him not to fill that one. As a result, I had a relapse within days.

My kids were not around to care for me. My ex-husband had flown up from Florida to Los Angeles to spend Christmas through New Years with the kids (my son had moved to California by then), and I was excluded from their celebrations, as my ex and I could not be in the same room. A friend of mine flew in to visit me on New Year's Day and beyond, but within days, I was back in the psych hospital again. Stopping the medication that would have interacted with my antinausea meds had been a mistake. The withdrawal had caused a rapid relapse.

My friend came to see me in the hospital once and was very kind. There was no embarrassment. She treated me like I was "not feeling well" and would be better very soon. I was. I didn't see her again before she went home.

I realized the error of not telling my surgeon I'd had previous adverse reactions to anesthesia. I should have found out which kinds were used in that original colostomy surgery, years before. I'd had other surgeries without insanity resulting, between that operation and the last one. Now I know not to fail to disclose the class of drugs that are dangerous to my mental health.

But those three episodes I've described are the only times I've ever had any sort of departure from sanity and lucidity. Following the last one, I was on psych meds for a number of months. Tranquilizers were involved. During that interlude, I was unable to continue working on my anal cancer book. I was unable to formulate complete sentences, let alone arrange them in a fashion that would entertain or inspire my readers, or fill them with delight at my cleverness, wit, and creativity. I would not have successfully convinced anyone that cancer could be survived, that life with cancer could be enjoyed, or that they, themselves, could be inspiring to others, if they were to, like me, be diagnosed with this scourge. I could barely answer a direct question coherently.

It was necessary to tell my psychiatrist that my liver was being damaged—and it was—by the combination of my chemotherapy and my psychiatric meds. That disclosure persuaded him to realize he was not improving or extending my life but was rather shortening it by keeping me medicated. My health and my disposition, in addition to my vocabulary and my intelligence, returned with vigor once the horrific medicines were removed from my daily regimen.

I regained my personality, and my disposition was greatly improved.

I've continued on various treatments for cancer, and it has been at times stable, and at times, it has progressed. But I have never again returned to a state of mania or depression. I have never again required psychiatric care.

Subsequently, my doctors determined that the episodes were very "normal" for patients in cancer treatment or following surgical procedures. It is because this doctor and others have assured me these events are "perfectly normal" that I decided to share my story.

Those experiences felt, at the time, anything but normal. I felt like a freak. A lunatic. A weirdo.

And if I feel like that at times, surely there are others. There have been many timidly asking if others with cancer in my support groups have needed psychiatric meds, whether mood stabilizers, antidepressants, or tranquilizers. I shared in hopes of making people feel that they, too, are "normal."

It is "normal" to have a severe emotional response to being diagnosed with a killer disease. It is "normal" to feel emotionally or mentally out of control, at times. It's normal to need someone to talk to. It's normal, at times, to need medications to help us feel more centered or "together" or "stable."

My initial "brief, reactive psychosis," as the psychiatrist diagnosed it, was due to a combination of my sensitivity to Vicodin and the shock of receiving a diagnosis of advanced cancer. To me, being told I had cancer was the same as if I'd been told, "You're going to die."

You may have that same, mind-numbing terror as a response to your cancer diagnosis. But as a friend told me then, I'll assure you, you are not in imminent danger of death. Probably. I mean, I'm no doctor, but what my friend told me has helped to this day. It was, "In your mind, you have to determine that you are going to live. Decide to live, and your mind will overrule your fear of death."

Obviously, like everyone else, we will eventually die, someday, of something. It's normal. Predictable, even. It's a part of life. I'm over the horror that cancer and pain are a part of my life. I sometimes have such severe pain that I can imagine someday, perhaps, welcoming death as a relief from pain and suffering. But eight years into my cancer experience, I'm seeing a pain specialist, and I'm getting the best relief I can find.

Your experience may not be like mine. Many people go into long-term remission. Some never have a recurrence of their cancer. It didn't work that way for me. I was "cancer free" for over a year after all my treatments, but then I had a recurrence in another location in my body of the same type of cancer. Spreading of the primary cancer is known as "metastasis."

I had surgery and chemo and was rid of all signs of cancer again for a year or two, but I had another metastasis. That time, some errors were made by some doctors, and I wasn't treated promptly for the third metastasis. As a result, the battle has been more difficult than it might have been. I've had "stability," meaning cancer remained but didn't grow or spread further, for a number of years. But I have not had more recurrences of "insanity" or "mania" or "delirium" or any number of labels that have been applied to my three episodes of temporarily losing control of my mind and my emotions. I have to admit, while it's distressing to battle a killer disease, I am greatly relieved to be doing it with all my mental faculties intact. My kids no longer have to fear that I'm lost to them forever, or developing Alzheimer's, or any of the other worries they confronted when I was not "in my right mind."

I'm sorry I cannot explain or even very acutely remember the depths of insanity that I experienced, but . . . the mind must handle many things . . . and "handling" news that you have a disease that may kill you is a tall order for the strongest and soundest of minds. My psyche has endured many things . . . a rape at age 19, three murder attempts by an escaped convict at age 21 . . . things that would drive a weaker person thoroughly insane. So a little thing like cancer should not have driven me nuts. It's likely, therefore, that the common denominator in all three instances is to blame: a class of drugs common to the pain medications and the anesthesia drugs that now appear on my drug allergy list.

Three surgical procedures following the use of Percocet and Vicodin and using a particular twilight sleep anesthesia. Three times I awoke in some kind of waking dream, in which the reality I was living starkly differed from the lunacy perceived by my loved ones and the strangers who dared to assess my mental condition. Three times I needed medication to bring me to my senses. My kids got me help. It worked. I have my mind back. They have their mom back.

You can come back from episodes of insanity brought on by drugs. And apparently, some people undergo depression or brief psychotic breaks as a result of experiencing trauma. Cancer and all its attending horrors lead many to describe themselves as suffering from PTSD, Post-traumatic Stress Disorder. More than one person has experienced those types of disturbances to their emotional health. But if this happens to you, it matters very little what sort of "label" the "experts" decide to apply to your condition. What you should understand is that as FREAKISH as it feels to "go nuts" for a while, it is "normal" to be emotionally shaken by the announcement that you have a disease that sometimes kills some people. Breakthroughs in treatment options are beginning to change the statistics, but the reality is that many people diagnosed with cancer WILL die. For that reason, it is extremely important to seek out the best doctors and the best care, whether for any psychiatric disturbance you may have or for cancer itself. The outcome of your cancer treatment relies heavily on the knowledge and skill of your doctors and your access to the latest treatment protocols and clinical trials.

What happened to my mind was fleeting and temporary. The ravages of cancer have been devastating, and many physical changes have been permanent. These are the things I should have feared more than the prospect of an early death. But even if temporary, losing my mind was more upsetting than most of the physical symptoms and changes. If you have had to take mood stabilizers or antidepressants or talk with a therapist during the course of your diagnosis and treatments, you should feel reassured. You are not a freak. You are normal. Thoughts may race, and feelings may swing like a pendulum wildly from one extreme to another. You haven't lost your mind. Just hold on to it; ask for help, and get your old self back. Or get a better self. Be a better version of yourself. If you are reading this because a mental disorder has affected your loved one with cancer, please get them help. Medications got me stable again, and I've enjoyed most of my eight years of life with and without cancer.

Also helpful are many online support groups. You'll find many on Facebook and elsewhere on the Internet, and you'll encounter hundreds, even thousands, experiencing many of the same difficulties you or your loved ones have faced. Make friends of a few or many of these people. It will help you to feel less alone and more normal. In many cases, deep friendships result, and emotional support from others is very valuable.

I have found myself receiving all manner of notes from people proclaiming that I have "inspired" them just by sharing my thoughts and feelings about cancer and about the symptoms I have had. You will find it very helpful to gain a sense of purpose that develops as you share your experiences with others. You will inspire many. I didn't expect to hear that I'm an "inspiration" to others. But it happened.

For eight years, I've survived in spite of having cancer. And I expect to one day hear that I'm cured. I hope you also will one day hear that you are completely free of cancer. Soon. And forever. Never ever let a potentially deadly diagnosis push you over the edge. See a therapist if you think you'll need one before you get the colonoscopy. Get prepared. Don't let it throw you. Fear is normal. But don't let it control you. Cancer can be beaten. You're going to be all right. Determine that you are going to live and savor every moment of your life, every moment with people you love. Loving others ultimately makes everything bearable. I wish you all the best.

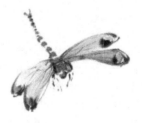

Chapter 15

When a Close Friend has Cancer

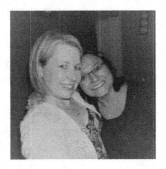

Sheila Roy
with Lynda Sie Greaves and Maureen Warren

ow do I even begin to write about something that is so difficult and can have so many endings? With a cancer diagnosis, we are left wondering if it will be ending one or ending two. I am writing this to talk about my friend, confidante, and kindred spirit Angela. I am writing this knowing she came out of this okay, but I am also writing from a place of grief as I lost my sweet mother recently. This loss has left me feeling like the emotional vault is open, and I can speak truly from a place in my heart.

We will also hear from Maureen and Lynda, other close friends of Angela. They will also share some of their experiences, feelings, thoughts, and advice regarding when a close friend is "walking" this ordeal we call cancer.

"Close friends share experiences, thoughts, feelings, secrets, dreams, fears, and challenges. When we fall, these special friends pick each other up, dust each other off, and face the uncharted path together, wishfully thinking that this friend is always going to be there. People who have this kind of friendship are blessed." - Maureen

The Dreaded Diagnosis That Changed Everything

The same day Angela had her colonoscopy, my son Liam was undergoing traumatic knee surgery for an injury he got while snowboarding. Angela was going for her appointment; "It will be fine," I told myself. I then focused on my son, who was in the operating room. The day went by, and I finally had the chance to text Angela to see how the test went. I received no reply, which is out of character for my friend. "She must be busy," I told myself.

A few hours later, I got the answer from her via text. "I can't talk now; I will call when I can." A feeling of cold dread ran through me, and I knew . . . I knew something was wrong. Angela, being the upbeat person that she is, always found a way of looking at the positive, but I still felt that pending phone call looming over me, as if the instant I answered it, our lives would change.

She called in the evening and broke the news to us she had anal cancer, stage 3, and that she was in a state of shock. She had so many people in her family and close friends to tell that she decided to write a blog online.

Worry and Fear Set In

I felt terrified and hollow. How could this be happening? Is this real? And how could this happen to someone so honest, kind, wonderful, and helpful to everyone?

"Hearing from my close friend that she had recently received an anal cancer diagnosis was devastating first and foremost for my friend. It was also difficult for the person who receives the news: me. If you have had past experience with cancer either in your family or personally, it can be overwhelming

142

and frightening. No prior experience with cancer can also make the announcement terrifying. This diagnosis came on the heels of both my friend and me losing our mothers-in-law to cancer within a year of each other. I remember feeling like I couldn't breathe, like I had been kicked in the stomach, and I couldn't get my breath, but I didn't let on about it." –Maureen

"This dreaded diagnosis came as a terrible blow. As Angela struggled to deal with this, as well as all its implications and anticipated treatments, so did family and friends. Among them, as her friend, I thought, "How can this happen? Angela is my healthy, vibrant, wonderful friend, who conscientiously takes care of herself. She eats well, goes to the gym, doesn't smoke, etc., so how can this happen to her?" Then, selfishly, came the thought, "What will I do if I lose my friend?" As the reality of the diagnosis sank in, I realized Angela was in for the battle of her life. As her friend, I thought what can I do? How can I help her as she goes to war against 'Cancer Up the Wazoo'?" –Lynda

I would read her blog posts, and the brutal honest details were really hard to read. I felt so sorry for what she and her family were going through. The post which stood out to me the most was the brutally honest truth of all the symptoms she was having and how much pain she was in.

"In her private blog, Angela says, 'I'm not a fighter. It's not in my nature to fight.' So crushing was the blow of the diagnosis, she says she isn't sure if she wants to live. This shocks me, as I know how much she loves life. On thinking about what she has said, I realize these thoughts are likely part of grieving that one's assumed excellent health is gone for the time being, and in its place is a large tumor that needs to be 'kicked in the butt.'" –Lynda

I visited her often in the weeks around the time of her diagnosis. She started going to many appointments as she was preparing for chemotherapy and radiation therapy. I bought her a rosary bracelet, and she wore it with so much faith.

I was very worried and truly wondered how this would all pan out. We had known each other for so many years. Our husbands also became good friends, and we would do things together as couples. Our children had also become good friends, like cousins. I spoke to my husband about how my closest friend was fighting for her life. He reassured me that she would be fine, but I could tell in his eyes he was very worried as well. He was concerned about her husband Agapito, also known as Cupp, and he said that the road ahead would be tough, as he had seen other people go through radiation and chemotherapy.

"I have a journal, and I wrote in it to vent my fears and hopes. To me, it was important to remain upbeat, hopeful, and positive, as well as remaining discreet." –Maureen

While Angela was going through the tests, diagnosis, and early days of treatment, we would attend Novena mass at the local Catholic church. Novena is a nine day or nine week period of public or private prayer to obtain special graces or favors. It was a comforting experience, but it also made the situation scarier when I realized we were there because of a very serious illness. That false bravado was weakening in me, and I was scared. I didn't really talk to anyone about how I was feeling because I am an avoider, and if I didn't talk about it, it didn't exist. Not a very healthy way to deal with a problem.

"Faith, prayer, and church are important to both my friend and me. When she asked me to go to a special Novena service with her and her family, my husband and I went. I prayed with her, and for her, and I prayed for myself too. There is power in prayer! I didn't want to lose my friend! We've been friends for so long now that I don't even know what I would do without her. We went to church together a few times over the course of the treatment, and I found it meaningful, uplifting, and peaceful." –Maureen

"Within the first few weeks post-diagnosis, I saw Angela turning to her faith. She invited her loved ones to attend church with her, which we did. We sang and prayed together, asking God for healing and support. I saw that faith was providing great comfort to Angela, and to all of us as well.

144

The church I attend has a prayer shawl ministry. Parishioners knit prayer shawls, which are blessed in church and given to others. I decided to knit a prayer shawl for Angela. I knit the shawl in a three-stitch seed pattern, which, in this ministry, was selected as symbolic of planting peace, healing, love, comfort, and hope. I chose colors that have certain attributes associated with them. These included aqua for courage and blue for healing and spirituality. Once I determined I would knit a shawl, I knitted fervently, with the goal of giving it to Angela before she began her treatment plan. Happily, I managed it. Angela loved it, and I believe it served to encircle her with feelings of love and support. My knitting is never perfect, but she didn't mind!" –Lynda

One evening, Angela and I and our husbands went for a drive to the park. We went for a nice long walk, but it was sad and morose, as our lives had changed. What seemed important a week prior was totally irrelevant now. Conversations that were not about life or death seemed shallow. My problems seemed so petty and small. Angela had bought a little stuffed lamb she named Hope, and she showed it to us that day. When we got home from our walk, all four of us cried. It was a scary, surreal moment.

Being a Supportive Friend During Treatment

Angela started her chemotherapy and radiation therapy in June. I went to visit her a few days after treatment started, and the Angela I saw was positive but tired and scared. She was lying down, so I crawled onto the bed and lay with her, all the while staring at her face. Her daughter Simone came in and lay on the bed, and we silently looked at each other with worry in our eyes. Angela looked small, pale, scared, and so tired. She was wearing her pajamas and had to get up to go to the bathroom every ten minutes, which looked like a huge chore for her. I was scared, worried, and felt so sorry for her.

Angela is always the upbeat, strong one in our group, and if she was scared, well, that made me terrified. I held her hand, and she slept and kept opening up her eyes to look at me. We didn't say much; we just looked into each other's eyes. I can remember that moment so clearly in my mind. It was a real integral moment for us, as I knew my friend would need me more than anything in the days to come.

"I treated her with new comfy pajamas because I knew she was spending a lot of time in bed. We saw movies together and enjoyed a girls' evening with other hometown friends."
—Maureen

As the weeks went on, the chemotherapy and radiation treatments were taking their toll on Angela. I was not able to talk to her that much. She was exhausted and doing her best to get through the day. I felt like I didn't want to bother her or disturb her. I felt that my day-to-day problems were not worthy to talk about, as they seemed shallow and trivial. How could I talk about my work, children, and other events, when my friend is battling cancer? I stopped talking about my life and what was going on in it, but in hindsight, I should have continued being the friend I already was and not change.

"I want to help and support Angela, but I don't know how. I've never been close to a family member or friend with a life-threatening cancer diagnosis. With my nursing background and being somewhat familiar with cancer and its treatment, I still feel ill-equipped to help her and somewhat helpless. I try to imagine how she must feel . . . I worry I won't find the right words to say to her, and then realize that none are adequate. On thinking about this, I conclude that to provide effective support and help to Angela, I must be guided by her and watch for her cues." —Lynda

As the days went on, Angela was showing signs of pain, fatigue, nausea, and sadness. I tried so hard to cheer her up and to say the right thing, but the only thing she really needed was rest and time. Angela was losing weight and looked so pale. My friend was in so much turmoil, yet there was nothing I could do. It was such a helpless feeling. My husband would always call Angela's husband and give him words of encouragement. As the weeks went on, it was nothing more than a waiting game.

"Again, I felt helpless. I watched for cues from Angela. I could see she felt supported and comforted by others' comments on

her blog, emails, phone calls, and short visits when possible."
–Lynda

I remember asking Angela if there was anything I could do for her that I was not doing already. Her answer was always, "No, you are doing everything I need at this time." When I look back at how many times I asked her this question, I realized I felt I was not doing enough. I felt like I could be doing more and be a better friend. I racked my brain for ideas of what I could do, say, or bring to her home (banana bread for the family was my go to). Truly, just being there for her was all she wanted, but it made me feel helpless at times. I have come to realize these feelings are normal, and when you care about someone so much, you want to take those feelings of hurt and pain away.

"Once I had the information I needed, I had to just follow my friend's lead in a supportive and constructive way. If she asked for something, I tried my best to do it. I made a point of seeing her more often when it was convenient for her. I also tried to back off the cancer talk unless it was important for her to share. I felt it was important to give her the opportunity to talk about what she was going through, but also the stuff we always talk about: husbands, kids, family, and the future. The future was tricky because the outcome of a cancer diagnosis is uncertain, but the future can be three hours from now, tomorrow, or even 'when my treatment is done.' I was fortunate enough to take her to one of her appointments when she needed a ride." –Maureen

"I tried to offer meaningful support. I made a point of knowing days and times of medical appointments, meetings, and tests so I could let her know I would be 'walking' with her at those times . . . I called and sent emails to see how things were going. I felt somewhat limited in how to support her during the actual treatment period, as Angela mostly needed to rest with family at her side. Again, for me, that created a helpless feeling . . . Having turned to her faith, Angela asked family and friends to pray for her, which I did. She found great comfort in this." –Lynda

In July, our daughter Mya got engaged to her boyfriend, Nick. It was such exciting news. Angela was so happy and excited for them, but the elephant in the room was would she be okay when the wedding took place? I was so worried at how I could share in the joy of my daughter knowing Angela was battling for her life. It was such a strange feeling, being so happy on the one hand, yet so scared and skeptical on the other. Our whole family had mixed feelings, happiness with a bit of a cloud above us. Cupp was so positive about his wife, but we could see the toll the worry was taking on him. He became a bit more quiet and pensive. We didn't want to think about the times ahead.

At the end of July, my family and I went on vacation, and we were informed that Angela had become very ill and had to be hospitalized. We were away, and my friend was sick and in the hospital. I was so worried and prayed every night for her life to become pain-free and for her to heal. How could this ever get better? I kept in contact with her son Lorenzo, and he told me she was quite ill, but he would keep me posted.

"I found it scary when my friend was hospitalized because she had come through all of those treatments and devastation with such strength and determination. I had never seen her in the hospital before. I couldn't understand the magnitude of damage radiation and chemotherapy do to all cells by reading about it in a book or a blog. The uncertainty came back. Is she going to be okay? Please God, don't let me lose my friend! . . . I also thought, 'How can I help other family members?' Her husband is Italian and one of the best cooks I know, so there is no way I could cook for them. I could, however, pick her mom up in our hometown, saving her husband travel time and helping out her mom too. Sometimes when you're sick, you just want Mom! I had an excellent road trip with her mom, making me feel closer still to my friend." –Maureen

By the time we came home from our holidays, Angela was out of the hospital but very immunocompromised. I had caught a cold, and I thought if I couldn't see her, we could at least talk on the phone. She was fatigued and weak, so our phone calls were only 5-10 minutes at the maximum.

"Sometimes I was unable to see my friend. It may have been my work and family commitments, complications from treatments, or a cold. I am a Kindergarten teacher, so I am regularly exposed to vast quantities of germs, which is not good for someone going through chemotherapy and radiation. For that matter, there are many reasons why we couldn't get together, even when we were both feeling well. At those times telephoning, texting, or FaceTiming to let her know I was thinking of her was helpful. I also read her personal blog, which kept me informed and gave me some insight as to what she was going through." –Maureen

Waiting for Results of Treatment

In August, Angela finally finished all her treatments. We were happy but worried at the same time. A doctor told her one of the most difficult waiting periods is the time between the end of treatment and when you get the final scan results to determine if the treatments have worked. Angela told me you don't want to have your scan too soon, as it may show residual tumor as the radiation still works on eliminating it for a few weeks even after treatment is over. Also, you don't want to wait too long because you are so worried and concerned about the results. Such a hard time, the waiting game, as we call it.

"During her recovery period, I was able to go to a few appointments with her, take tea over for a short visit, etc. I felt good that I could help more actively, but tried to watch for cues from her that would tell me how long I should stay, what she wanted to talk about—to be sensitive to whether she felt like discussing her illness, or just chatting in light conversation . . . . Severe side effects of treatment persisted and would do so indefinitely. I could see that, in facing this reality, Angela felt deflated and somewhat depressed. I found this difficult, being unaccustomed to her feeling like this. Again, I watched for cues, and Angela was comfortable to say whether she felt like talking or a visit." –Lynda

In that time, I went from believing she was cured to worrying and praying the awful cancer was gone from her body. My mindset totally changed from what *was* important to what truly *is* important.

While we were waiting for news of the final scan and post-treatment tests, we didn't talk about it very much. I was almost too scared to ask. In fact, I did not even know the date of the final scan until a few weeks before. The feelings I had waffled between fear and anger this was happening to someone so kind, to disbelief and utter sadness for what had transpired and what was to come.

What I Have Learned

This experience has left me feeling I can help others who are going through something similar. I think the most important thing is to be there for whenever they want to talk or be there when they just need a warm hand to hold. I think the hardest thing is telling yourself there is no right thing to say or do to make the person feel better. You just have to be there with them and feel the experience, to not try to solve the problem, but to be positive and nurturing.

I remember Angela sharing with me that people were telling her about the experiences they went through with loved ones who had cancer and some of the negative outcomes. I remember her saying all she wanted was positivity and strength, and the negative stories understandably brought her down. There are so many positive outcomes when people are diagnosed with cancer, and we need to focus on those and give the hope that this disease can be cured. Without hope, we have nothing. So if I can give or share one truly very important thing, it is to be positive and believe in one's heart that people can be healed.

The experience Angela went through has changed me considerably. I feel that many of the things I worried about before are not so important at this time. The worries that bothered me have become insignificant. It really has put things into perspective for me and has made me realize health is the biggest wealth in the world. We tend to take things for granted until something affects us personally. We think we are somehow spared, but in truth, it has taught me life is so very fragile, and we need to realize the gift we have been given.

"I have a much greater understanding of the impact of a life-threatening cancer diagnosis on patient, family, and friends. I've had a front row seat to witness the grief, pain, and body changes that go along with it . . . At my stage in life, I know the value of friendship. However, this experience reinforced how very precious close friends are, and that friendship mustn't be taken for granted, for we don't know what lies ahead . . . I learned to support; you mustn't worry about saying or doing the right thing. If you watch for the cues given by the one you are trying to support, you can't go wrong."
—Lynda

Normalcy Again

I am so truly thankful to God and to the medical field and research that has helped my friend recover from this disease. It's a long road to recovery, as she has shared with me. But it's been a whirlwind of emotion to come to the place we are at. Normalcy—that's a beautiful word. I love the fact that we are talking about hairstyles, books, movies, and things we have always talked about. We are going out on double dates again, and we are not living in the fear we did a year ago.

"Thankfully, this period passed, and Angela is much better in every way. I was thrilled when she shared that treatment was successful. As her doctor said to her—'You've won your battle!' She met her goal, which was to 'Kick Cancer In The Butt.'"
—Lynda

It is now back to the point where my dear friend is helping me with some of the issues I am dealing with now with the loss of my mother. She is helping me with my dad who is coping with the loss of his wife of 66 years. Angela is back in full force, and as wonderful, positive, and loving as ever, and I am forever grateful for that. I could not live without her—and I won't have to.

"Anal Cancer and the damage it does aren't over when you hear the No Evidence of Disease news from your friend. We're still healing! Counseling, rehab, getting back to work and normalcy are just some of the hurdles we face. We can suffer from depression and anxiety. What if the cancer comes back?

Listen to your friend, love, be there when you're needed, stay positive and be informed. Be the friend you would want to have! Live, love, and laugh!" –Maureen

"As Angela turned to her faith, so did I. I want to thank her for opening this door for me. As a result, I have become more active in my church's Prayer Shawl Ministry and another volunteer program. I enjoy attending church more regularly, and find great comfort there, as I know Angela did." –Lynda

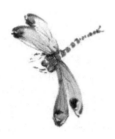

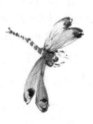

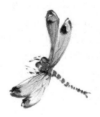

Chapter 16

Peripheral Neuropathy

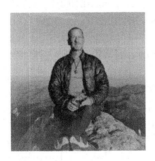

An Interview with Michael DeHart

Michael DeHart has been diagnosed with cancer for the second time. He has been living with peripheral neuropathy for many years, and he was interested in sharing what he knows in hopes of helping others who may be living with this condition. Following is an interview I had with him. He is currently facing treatment for anal cancer.

Angela G. Gentile: *Can you explain what peripheral neuropathy (PN) is in an easy-to-understand way?*

Michael DeHart: Peripheral neuropathy is caused by damage to your peripheral nerves–most frequently in your hands and feet. Peripheral neuropathy varies significantly in severity, ranging from mildly annoying but relatively easily controlled to debilitating pain and neurological damage that can impair mobility and motor skills. It can be caused by many factors, including metabolic and endocrine disorders (diabetes being a prime example), autoimmune disorders, HIV medications, infections, heavy alcohol consumption, vitamin B12 deficiency, cancers themselves, and chemotherapy drugs used to treat cancers. Peripheral neuropathy is also fairly common—about 20 million Americans have some degree of peripheral neuropathy. (Mayo Clinic online has more information you may want to check out.)

Basically, it feels like burning, unpleasant tingling, weakness, and/or numbness. Peripheral neuropathy can be short-term or permanent, with short-term neuropathy generally resolving in a few months to a few years at most. Severe peripheral neuropathy (which is what I have) is often permanent. That being said, there are medications and tricks for learning how to deal with it!

When and why did you get it?

In 1996, I had non-Hodgkin's lymphoma and underwent six cycles of CHOP chemotherapy (cyclophosphamide, doxorubicin, vincristine, and prednisone), which saved my life, so anal cancer is not my first trip to the dance floor with cancer. CHOP, while highly effective in treating non-Hodgkin's lymphoma, is a beast regarding side effects. For me, the most lasting (22 years later) is peripheral neuropathy. Peripheral neuropathy is a relatively common side effect of chemotherapy, though the rate of occurrence varies dramatically depending on what chemotherapy drugs a patient is given.

Mitomycin (Mitomycin-C), one of the most common first-line chemotherapy drugs for anal cancer (usually given in combination with 5-FU) is known to cause peripheral neuropathy in some anal cancer patients (though in a minority number of cases, less than 20%). Cisplatin is another chemotherapy drug used to treat anal cancer and is often given to anal cancer patients who present with more advanced disease (stage 3 or 4). Those who receive chemotherapy regimens including cisplatin are much more likely to experience peripheral neuropathy than those who receive mitomycin.

What are some of the symptoms?

When I first developed peripheral neuropathy during the time I had lymphoma, there were many days I could not walk to the mailbox and back. Tingling and burning sensations were terrible, but for me, the worst was that about every minute or so the nerves in my feet would be on fire, and this horrible, burning/throbbing sensation would be sent all the way up my legs—sometimes severe enough to make me gasp and take my breath away. I'd lie there and curl up into the fetal position for hours. It was so bad, I required opioid drugs in order to dull the pain. I would also drop glasses and plates left and right, fumble with keys when opening a door, and forget all about being able to type or text well. My grip strength lessened, and it was emotionally difficult as it so physically limited me for an extended period.

As peripheral neuropathy most frequently affects the hands or feet (particularly the feet), it can be very frustrating doing basic activities such as walking, opening doors, turning a key in a lock, etc.—actions that most of us take for granted. It can make it challenging to feel things, and because of this, it's tough to judge how firmly you need to grasp things in order not to drop them. Peripheral neuropathy also flares up most commonly in the evening, which can make it very difficult to sleep. In fact, many people with mild to moderate peripheral neuropathy don't notice it until it's bedtime.

What do you do to manage it?

Gabapentin (Neurontin) is the most common medication to treat peripheral neuropathy and is part of the regimen I use to manage neuropathy. Unfortunately for me, as my neuropathy was severe, I was on the highest dosage regularly given of gabapentin (5.4g/day— I was taking six 300mg pills in the morning and twelve at night!). The problem for me is that such a high dose of gabapentin made me a total space cadet—my memory was shot; I would physically shake. It made me clumsy, and I could not think clearly. I'm a statistician and entrepreneur by trade, so not being able to think clearly was a huge problem for me.

Sometimes, antidepressant medicines are used to treat peripheral neuropathy because many people seem to benefit from them. I've been put on duloxetine (Cymbalta), and it has been a game changer. Duloxetine in doses lower than that used to treat depression is often effective for neuropathy. I currently take 900mg of gabapentin at night and 30mg of duloxetine. I tried to take 60mg of duloxetine and no gabapentin, but for me, the 60mg dose of duloxetine had too many undesirable side effects.

It's been a lengthy trial and error process, but my neuropathy is now relatively well-controlled. I do have breakthrough neuropathy sometimes (ironically, I'm having that shooting pain in my left foot as I'm working on this!), but finding the right balance of medications has been life-changing. I'm now an avid athlete—long-distance hiker, backpacker, and rock and mountain climber—all activities that are hard on the feet.

Does it hold you back in any way?

Not really. I won't lie—the occasional night still happens where I have real problems due to extremely painful throbbing in my feet. Sometimes it lasts for a few hours. When it does, I turn on the TV, take an extra dose of gabapentin, and just try to deal with it. But I refuse to let it rule me, and I refuse not to have a positive attitude about it. It would be nice not to have to take gabapentin or duloxetine, but it's an acceptable price to pay for a much higher quality of life than I'd have otherwise.

Talk a little bit about your new diagnosis of anal cancer and any concerns you have about PN and anal cancer.

I've recently been diagnosed with anal cancer; at this point, I'm very lucky it appears to be stage 1. I am concerned about what mitomycin may do in terms of exacerbating my already existing neuropathy. It's always a concern when a patient has existing neuropathy, and they must be given more chemotherapy drugs. I've had my share of health concerns—I've been HIV positive for 27 years, survived non-Hodgkin's lymphoma, had a partial discectomy (partial removal of one of the discs in my spine), had spinal fusion surgery, prior anal intraepithelial neoplasia (AIN) ablation surgery, etc.—but through it all I've been positive and optimistic. During all this I've gotten a Bachelor's degree in Mathematics, an MBA, started companies in the US and Africa, and been quite athletic and fit. My biggest concern, other than surviving anal cancer (which is expected in my case), is my neuropathy may return with a vengeance and require opioid drugs to control if it gets too out of hand. For me, that would be significantly emotionally difficult as it could limit physical activities I love such as rock climbing as well as impair my mental abilities, which are critical for the type of profession I have.

What advice do you have for those who may have peripheral neuropathy?

Learn to be tough. Decide that you ARE going to have a normal life, with or without neuropathy, period. Learn what works for you concerning medical management—many people don't require anything near the maximum dose of gabapentin that I required for neuropathy control so your journey with it may be easier than mine. It may require a combination of medications, but don't give up! Also, it may go away on its own, so stay optimistic.

I think it's imperative to stay as physically active as you can, as so much of the battle with any chronic pain condition is depression. Do what you can. Walk ten steps today if that's all you can manage and try for 11 tomorrow and 12 the day after that. Eventually, ten steps will become the ability to walk to your mailbox and back, and soon you'll be walking around the block. I've gone from being unable to walk to the mailbox to a 20-mile hike in a day. Stay committed to doing your best, and you will learn how to manage your neuropathy.

In addition to trying to stay as physically active as you can, eat a healthy diet and maintain a healthy weight to the best of your ability. In particular, make sure you get plenty of vitamin B12 in your diet or take B12 supplements as B12 deficiency can increase your risk for neuropathy. Good sources of B12 include fish, poultry, meat, milk, and yogurt. Plant sources are not good sources of vitamin B12, and even organizations such as The Vegan Society acknowledge that the only good vegan sources of B12 come from foods that are fortified with B12 (such as some breakfast cereals) or nutritional yeast. Obesity has also been linked to neuropathy, and even if it doesn't cause neuropathy, more weight on your feet will cause more pain.

Can you share any useful resources you have found?

The most important resource is your medical team, particularly your oncology team and your primary care physician. New techniques are coming out, such as wearing "frozen gloves and socks" to help reduce chemotherapy-induced peripheral neuropathy.

Sooner rather than later, let your doctors know if you experience any peripheral neuropathy symptoms, as oncologists have a very high level of knowledge concerning how to help you manage your neuropathy.

The Foundation for Peripheral Neuropathy (*foundationforpn.org*) is a public charity foundation that serves as an excellent resource across a wide range of topics ranging from education to treatment information to finding the latest peripheral neuropathy clinical trials. If you are newly diagnosed with neuropathy, the Foundation for Peripheral Neuropathy can also help you find a local support group.

Thanks, Michael! And all the best to you as you go into treatment for anal cancer.

You're welcome.

****

RESOURCES:

Mayo Clinic. "Peripheral Neuropathy." https://www.mayoclinic.org/diseases-conditions/peripheral-neuropathy/symptoms-causes/syc-20352061. Retrieved 03 Sep 2018.

The Foundation for Peripheral Neuropathy
(*foundationforpn.org*)

Chapter 17

Integrative Medicine: The Ultimate Holistic Approach to Cancer Care

Angela G. Gentile

A study released in 2017 found that people who forgo standard medical treatment for their common and curable cancer are more than twice as likely to die within five years (Johnson, Park, Gross & Yu). So I ask, why are people still choosing alternative medicine and forgoing conventional treatments like chemotherapy, radiation therapy, and hormone treatments? In this chapter, we explore this topic and examine what may be the best approach to treating cancer—that being an integrative one.

When faced with a cancer diagnosis, many thoughts go through the mind. A typical reaction is, "Will I survive this? Am I going to die?" Considering today's conventional medicine and technological advances, it is possible the person will survive, depending on how advanced the cancer is. If they catch it early enough, there is a higher chance of survival. Add some safe, complementary therapies that don't interfere with the conventional treatment, and we have what I call the best of both worlds—Integrative Medicine.

Cancer causes a feeling of loss of control in its victim. The person's body is attacking itself, and that attack could prove fatal. The thoughts of death and loss of the future, future pain or possible disfigurement, and the prospect of cancer treatment side effects and how this will affect loved ones can heighten feelings of anxiety, worry, stress, grief, loss, fear, and panic, and can significantly affect one's overall sense of well-being. Mind-body connection activities like yoga (for caregivers and family members, too!) can help give a sense of control and peace and can help calm the mind and get the emotions in check. It provides a person with a sense of control.

Distress is so often caused by painful memories, guilt over things from the past, or anxieties regarding the future. Mindfulness and meditation can bring a person into the present moment. It has been proven that mind-body connection exercises increase quality of life and sense of well-being. Many of these therapies can work synergistically, meaning they have even more benefit when used together. The thought of meditation daunts some people as they imagine it calls for the concentration of the Buddha. But that is not so; there are many very approachable forms of meditation, and all can find a style that works for them.

In today's cancer world, there seem to be two camps. There are the "conventional medicine" folks and the "alternative medicine" camp. There are strong feelings and opinions on both sides. I have been involved in these kinds of debates. People who believe in alternative methods and medicines try to convince those who have cancer that "The Big Three" (chemotherapy, radiation therapy, and surgery) standard treatments are no more than poison, or "burn and slash," and they are not good for us. Added to the Big Three now are hormone therapy, immunotherapy (such as Keytruda), and targeted therapies including monoclonal antibodies and small molecule inhibitors such as Herceptin for Her2 breast cancer—so now it's the "Big Six" perhaps?

Those championing alternative medicines tend to believe there is a better and more natural way to cure cancer, and although they mean well, they may make the person who has considered the conventional route of treatment doubt themselves. The person who trusts the reported efficacy of standard treatment sometimes feels as though she or he has to try to convince the alternative folks that there is no evidence to prove their theory works. Many supporters of alternative treatment only will come back with all kinds of anecdotal (informal or unscientific) instances of how "someone's cancer was treated, and the person was cured" using, as examples, medical marijuana or Essiac® tea.

There are cases of survival (and death) on both sides. Some people survive cancer using standard treatment, and yes, some survive using unconventional approaches. The problem is we don't have scientific evidence to prove or disprove, for example, "medical marijuana cures all cancers" (because there are over 100 types of cancers). However, for example, we DO have evidence that Essiac® tea is NOT SCIENTIFICALLY PROVEN to treat or prevent cancer.

Cancer researcher/psychotherapist Kelly A. Turner, Ph.D. has studied the commonalities of people who experience a radical remission, and she has published a book that explains more about the nine key factors shared by most people who survive cancer. The *New York Times* bestseller by Turner, *Radical Remission, Surviving Cancer Against All Odds* (2014), reveals some intriguing information on these factors that can make a real difference.

These nine key remission factors are related to (in no particular order):

✓ taking control of your health (adopting an active role, embracing change, and conquering resistance),
✓ changing your diet,
✓ using herbs and supplements,
✓ following your intuition,
✓ clearing emotional blockages,
✓ increasing positive emotions,
✓ seeking social supports,
✓ embracing spiritual growth, and
✓ having strong reasons for living.

Turner believes most people will need "conventional medicine to outrun cancer." I found this book very encouraging and recommend it.

When I was diagnosed with anal cancer, I wanted to know what my options were. I spoke with an oncologist who told me the approach shown to be 70% effective for my type of cancer was called the Nigro Protocol. This was a chemoradiation approach, which did not include surgery. He said he wanted me to "keep all my parts." I felt fairly confident this was the way to go.

However, I still wanted to know if there was a gentler and kinder, more natural cure. My online research led me to discover a woman, Corrie Yelland, who states she has successfully used cannabis oil (marijuana) to treat her anal cancer. She explains that she had one diagnostic surgery and one biopsy. The doctors told her she would need to have radiation treatments. After researching what pelvic radiation could do to her, Corrie decided against it and turned to cannabis oil. She took it internally and topically–ingesting cannabis oil on a daily basis and inserting gelatin capsules filled with a mixture of the oil and olive oil into her anus (cannabis oil suppositories). She believes it has kept her alive and cured her of cancer. She also states, "I have helped coach quite a few others to an 'all clear' status with anal cancer . . . using only the oil." Cannabis oil is not an approved cancer treatment, and in some jurisdictions, it is still illegal to use.

I even arranged to have a talk with a cancer treatment clinic in Tijuana, Mexico. After reminding me some five times via email they would call me at 4:00 pm on a specified day, I didn't hear from them. I had gone on to do something else, then they called at 4:35 pm. I missed the call, and they never tried contacting me again.

I tried to find a more natural option to eliminate my squamous cell carcinoma but came up against a brick wall. The "secret" (only known to those who have a web link address) online anal cancer support group I was a member of supported me no matter what I decided, but they said the ladies who took the alternative route were no longer alive. Even the nurses and healthcare professionals in the group said the treatment was brutal, but no other option was scientifically proven to be more successful. Lamentably, when people pushing natural programs respond to people who have cancer in these casual, disorganized ways, it's difficult to take it seriously enough to feel confident about such alternatives.

I have concluded regarding these alternative therapy cancer clinics that they are perhaps helpful to those who have no other options or those who are willing to take a risk and try new and emerging treatment modalities which are not yet available to them locally or scientifically proven. If the doctor or specialists feel there is nothing more they can do (perhaps the cancer has spread too far) and the person wishes to pursue other options, then this is where these types of therapies come in. Treatments at these clinics may cost thousands of dollars, and they come with no guarantee, so it's a risk the person has to take (sadly, it's not only "Big Pharma" that wants to line their pockets).

People who have a late-stage case of cancer, incurable cancer, or are approaching the end of life can be very vulnerable to "snake oil" salespeople. Those offering a magic potion or elixir, appearing just at the right place at the right time, can easily convince a terrified, weakened, stressed, suffering person to hand over his or her cash in hopes of a miracle cure. Naïve and desperately hopeful people can easily fall prey to frauds, quacks, and charlatans. The website called Quackwatch (*quackwatch.org*) has an impressive listing of many types of health claims, and you can search for anything you have heard of to see what their researched take is on it.

We all want to believe there is a simple solution to cancer. We donate money, raise funds for, and even pray for a cure. Unfortunately, some believe in cancer conspiracy theories, that there is a "hidden cure," and doctors and pharmaceutical companies are holding it back for personal gain. Some believe there is more money to be made by the medical system by not releasing this supposed "cure" for cancer. Many point fingers at Big Pharma and spread malicious propaganda that there is a conspiracy against the general public, while at the same time selling their unproven, potentially unsafe "cures." Some feel the pharmaceutical industry is not working for the benefit of the people; instead, they are cashing in for their own benefit. I don't believe this to be true. If and when there is a cure for cancer (which means there would need to be many cures as there are many types) I am sure the researchers will rejoice and get a Nobel Prize! Hopefully, these cures are just around the corner.

Until then, we have to rely on what scientific research is telling us. Evidence-based solutions, those tested in labs and done objectively with proper research methods, are the best bet we have toward increasing our chances for a cure and our survival rates (living long with or after cancer). There is a group of researchers who go over all the scientific cancer studies that have been done and come up with an overall take on the situation. This group of scientists prepares "Cochrane Reviews." Many subjects can be found on their website (*cochrane.org*). For example, there were over 40 articles on "diet and cancer."

During my research investigations, I have come to realize the scientific studies must be looked at very carefully. For example, if a pharmaceutical company is providing the research grant (funding) to determine the efficacy (success) of one of their newest chemotherapy drugs, we can be sure if the results are favorable, we need to look carefully at how the study was done. This is true for any research. How many subjects were in the study? Were they randomly selected? Was it done as a double-blind study (neither participants or experimenters knew who had the treatment versus placebo)? Was there a control group (a group that received usual or standard care)? This is true for any research that may have a bias (favoring one side). This is also known as a conflict of interest. For example, if the study was funded by the pharmaceutical company that makes the drug, they will most likely be looking for favorable results. If the study was peer-reviewed, examined by other experts in the field, that's a big plus. You will see quality studies published in peer-reviewed journals. All of these factors must be taken into account when doing your research. For more on this, check out the article by Jeremy Adam Smith, "Ten Questions to Ask about Scientific Studies" (2015).

When others give suggestions of magic potions, they feel they are genuinely helping you in your journey to heal and overcome your illness. It eases their stress, providing a sense of some control over the situation and that of being helpful. We are all human, and we all want to feel in control; one of our primary instincts is to survive. We seek answers to why things happen and answers to our problems. Without those answers, we can feel vulnerable. Cancer makes us feel that way—unprotected—and it can greatly affect our mindset. If there is a "magic tea" to make you feel better, someone may suggest it. It is like handing over a package of hope and optimism. Hope helps us think positively about our future. Positive thinking can also help our bodies produce "feel-good" chemicals in the brain, to help us feel like everything is fine in the here and now. Naturally-produced hormones like serotonin, endorphins, and dopamine can help us feel better, while stress hormones like cortisol and adrenaline can cause hormonal imbalances, which can affect our mood and even our ability to meet physical challenges like illness. Reducing stress, improving our mindset, and engaging in distracting and meaningful activity can be beneficial to those affected by a cancer diagnosis, as they help reduce the body's stress hormones.

I remember one friend (whom I would consider in the alternative camp) gave me a box full of literature and videos on *The Truth About Cancer* and *Cancer: Step Outside of the Box* by Ty M. Bollinger. I was aware of this series before my diagnosis, and I truly believed if I ever got cancer, I wouldn't do the chemotherapy and radiotherapy route as it seemed too dangerous and came with risky side effects. I had already begun to be seduced by the rhetoric and fear-mongering. This friend also gave me a big chunk of turmeric (a plant of the ginger family) and told me to consider an apricot seed diet or one based on just carrots. These solutions seemed far too simple, and although I read some of the book and watched some of the videos, my scientific and practical intelligence woke up and steered me in the other direction. My gut feeling told me cancer was a beast, and diet alone could not cure it. If I wanted to live, I needed to bring out the big guns. This friend also wanted me to promise her if I ever got cancer again that I wouldn't do chemotherapy or radiation therapy. I couldn't.

I also remember a neighbor's friend who wanted to make sure I received information on how he treated cancer. He sent me an email with details on the "Budwig Protocol." They base it on a diet of primarily cottage cheese and high-quality fresh flaxseed oil. He shared a story about his dog, diagnosed with high-grade melanoma and treated successfully with this diet. He wanted me to do my research to see if the cottage cheese and flax seed oil diet may help me. I decided it wasn't for me.

I am sure people who provide others with these magic potions and miracle cures mean well. Unfortunately, for someone who is facing a cancer diagnosis, it can make one feel confused and uncertain. A person diagnosed with cancer is (most likely) already dealing with life and death decisions, and more doubt and fear can increase stress and anxiety. We all know stress and anxiety are not good for us as they can affect our natural hormones and brain chemicals as noted above.

Definitions of Cancer Treatment Approaches

In order to move forward with a basic understanding of different approaches and technologies for treating cancer, we must define what they mean. The online National Cancer Institute (NCI) Dictionary of Cancer Terms provides basic definitions for the next four terms.

Conventional medicine: A system in which medical doctors and other healthcare professionals (such as nurses, pharmacists, and therapists) treat symptoms and diseases using drugs, radiation, or surgery. Also called allopathic medicine, biomedicine, mainstream medicine, orthodox medicine, and Western medicine.

Standard medical care (or standard medical treatments): Treatments that are accepted by medical experts as a proper treatment for a specific type of disease, and are widely used by healthcare professionals. Also called best practice, standard of care, and standard therapy.

Alternative medicine: Treatments used instead of standard treatments. Standard treatments are based on the results of scientific research and are currently accepted and widely used. Less research has been done for most types of alternative medicine. Alternative medicine may include special diets, mega-dose vitamins, herbal preparations, special teas, and magnet therapy. For example, one may be on a special diet instead of anticancer drugs as a treatment for cancer.

Complementary medicine: Treatments used along with standard treatments, but not considered standard. Standard treatments are based on the results of scientific research and are currently accepted and widely used. Less research has been done for most types of complementary medicine. Complementary medicine includes acupuncture, dietary supplements, massage therapy, hypnosis, and meditation. For example, acupuncture may be used with certain drugs to help keep blood counts up and to lessen cancer pain, nausea, and vomiting.

Together, complementary and alternative treatments are usually referred to as CAM.

Integrative medicine (IM) is a type of medical care that combines conventional (standard) medical treatment with complementary and alternative (CAM) therapies that have been shown to be safe and to work. CAM therapies treat the mind, body, and spirit. In my opinion, this holistic approach is best when working toward healing, restoring and maintaining health.

The National Center for Complementary and Integrative Health (NICCIH) prefers to use the term "complementary health approaches" for non-standard care and "integrative health" when discussing the combination of mainstream healthcare combined with non-mainstream methods.

Complementary Health Approaches

There are three categories of complementary health approaches: 1. Natural products, 2. Mind and body practices, and 3. "Others." Natural products include dietary supplements such as herbs, vitamins, minerals, and probiotics. Mind and body practices include yoga, spirituality, chiropractic, meditation, and massage therapy. The third category comprises approaches that don't fit into either of the other two—traditional Chinese medicine, homeopathy, naturopathy, Ayurvedic medicine, and other traditional healing approaches.

A study published in 2000 found that almost all cancer patients attending an outpatient clinic in Texas, USA were aware of CAM, and at least 83% of them had used at least one CAM approach. Spiritual practices were used by 81%, vitamins and herbs used by 63%, and movement and physical therapies by 59%.

Risk Tolerance

Life comes with guaranteed risks. For example, walking out the door and crossing the street comes with a risk. We may not see that car or motorcycle and get hit. There may be a drunk driver behind the wheel. I am sure you can think of many other examples. Cancer treatment and risk tolerance is a very deep subject. Everyone has the right to choose their treatment regime and procedures whether or not others agree with it.

Standard care chemotherapy and radiation therapy come with risks. For example, chemotherapy can kill a person because it can affect the immune system to a point where it can't fight off infection anymore. Radiation therapy can cause "burns" (including sores and ulcers), which can cause infection. Surgery also comes with risks. Standard medical care is not accident-proof. Too much of this, too little of that, one slip and poof, disaster. People who are provided with these options must weigh out the risks against the benefits. Doctors and other specialists will discuss these risks and the likelihood of adverse outcomes.

There are over 250 anti-cancer or chemotherapeutic drugs listed on the National Cancer Institute's website. Many of these therapies are used in combination. On the website, each type of cancer comes with listed recommended therapies (although at time of printing there was none listed for anal cancer). These approved therapies have been through rigorous scientific studies and provide patients and healthcare professionals with a fair degree of confidence.

Radiation therapy has limited options. It is either administered from outside the body (external-beam), inside (brachytherapy), or systemic (through the blood). A radiation oncologist prescribes the dose intensity, frequency, and number of treatments.

Regarding alternative medicine options, there are hundreds, perhaps thousands for those who have cancer. These options also come with risks. For example, apricot seeds, also known as amygdalin, come with a risk of cyanide poisoning. Black Salve can corrode the skin. Coffee enemas have been linked to several deaths. Even though something seems natural, it doesn't mean it's safe. Consider this: The sub-Saharan African black mamba snake's venom is completely natural, but it can kill a human.

With all therapies, research is highly recommended. Speaking to a trusted healthcare professional or another qualified specialist will help allay any fears or questions one may have. Getting a second or third opinion is also recommended if you feel you need more reassurance. Each person's situation is different, so even if two people have the same cancer, their treatment protocol may be different.

We all come with different health histories, priorities, life stages, cancer profiles, and so much more. Where we live, whom we live with, etc. can also affect our course of treatment. I know a woman who wanted to be at her son's wedding, so she delayed her second round of chemo so she would feel well enough to attend.

Educating Ourselves is Key

I found a few websites and books on CAM, and I am educating myself continually on the subject. I have found a few CAMs I believe in and have used. Some are merely for the psychological benefit, and some are for the mind-body connection. For example, self-affirmations (see Appendix A) and prayer helped me through the most difficult times of my cancer ordeal.

The Canadian Cancer Society brochure called "Complementary Therapies: A guide for people with cancer" (2014) explains a lot more about what their position is on the subject. They include information on acupuncture, aromatherapy, art therapy, biofeedback, energy therapies (e.g., Therapeutic Touch, Reiki), guided imagery, hypnosis, massage therapy, meditation, music therapy, naturopathic medicine, tai chi, and yoga. I attended restorative yoga and art therapy programs the cancer center offered free of charge.

There is much to be said about the placebo effect. This is the mysterious phenomenon whereby if a person believes a treatment will help him or her, it most likely will. Many of the alternative therapies have been found to be nothing more than a placebo effect, and I have read two excellent books on the subject. One is called *Do You Believe in Magic? The sense and nonsense of alternative medicine* by Paul A. Offit, M.D. (2013), and the other is *Trick or Treatment? Alternative medicine on trial* by Simon Singh and Edzard Ernst (2008). They are eye-opening books. I believe if an alternative treatment is safe, doesn't cost too much (or free is better!), and it doesn't interfere with conventional treatment, then it's worth a try. The mind works in mysterious ways, and it's always a good idea to keep it open to new methods of healing and improving one's mindset. The placebo effect can do wonders. Interestingly, there was a study on people given a placebo (a pill with no medicine in it) for cancer-related nausea, and it helped more than the standard care group. They even knew they were getting a placebo!

I have found the Internet is full of "fake news" and unsubstantiated claims for many alternative treatments. I believe others are best helped by seeking valid, reliable, scientific information. A global search on the Internet can be overwhelming. In addition to searching medical journals in the online libraries such as PubMed and the National Institutes of Health (NIH), I have found two books that have been helpful. *The Desktop Guide to Complementary and Alternative Medicine: An evidence-based approach*, second edition, by editors Ernst, Pittler, and Wider (2006) has comprehensive and easy-to-read tables and charts to help one decide on what alternative and complementary therapies are potentially helpful as well as any safety risks associated with them. Physicians use this book, so the language can be daunting. The other book, which is easier to read and is also written for both those diagnosed with cancer and doctors, is the *American Cancer Society Complete Guide to Complementary and Alternative Cancer Therapies*, second edition (2009). I read through both regarding acupuncture, and they both indicate acupuncture shows positive results in helping relieve nausea and vomiting, especially for reducing the vomiting that can occur after chemotherapy.

There are some great forums and groups on the Internet where you can dialog with others who are interested in natural cures, cancer treatments, and other forms of holistic healing. If you are interested in this topic, do an Internet or Facebook search for a group that may suit your interests. I have found supportive and helpful groups on Facebook. Just make sure if you are considering a complementary treatment you research the benefits and risks. Ask yourself (and perhaps a trusted medical professional) is it safe, is it affordable, plus is it compatible with my conventional treatment?

Any vitamins, supplements, herbs, or any other special teas and diets a person with cancer is taking should be discussed with a doctor, nurse, or dietician. This especially applies to a person receiving chemotherapy or radiation therapy. I have read a lot about Gerson therapy and the Hoxsey diet (and there are many others), but I am not convinced these are safe or effective nutritional approaches to controlling or curing cancer. The Alkaline vs. Acidic diet is another one I hear about, which is based on avoiding foods that make your blood PH more acidic. Sometimes there isn't enough evidence either way to support or encourage the use of natural health products (like probiotics) or certain diets. So, it's best to advise your cancer care team about what you are taking.

Integrative medicine and its holistic approach to care is most effective toward treating cancer as it uses the best of both worlds. I know someone who saw both a medical oncologist and a naturopathic doctor at the same time. These doctors consulted with each other, and both agreed this woman needed chemotherapy, as her breast cancer was very aggressive. She is using that with some natural herbal products. Finding doctors and cancer clinics/hospitals open to both conventional and unconventional approaches to care is like hitting the jackpot. Improvements in treatment results, quality of life, hope, and comfort are what most people want.

If you are interested in attending a cancer center that incorporates integrative medicine, start by asking your doctor for a recommendation. You can also try searching the Internet for "integrative cancer center" and see what comes up. Find out what kinds of treatments are offered. For example, there may be access to spiritual care, peer guidance, or a support group. I am hopeful for the future of evidence-based, integrative care for those affected by cancer or other chronic illnesses. Closing the door to either conventional medicine or CAM will most likely mean you are missing out on some treatment and healing opportunities—for body, mind, and soul.

****

REFERENCES:

Ernst, E., Pittler, M. H. & Wider, B. (Ed.s) (2006). *The Desktop Guide to Complementary and Alternative Medicine: An evidence-based approach*, (2nd ed.). Philadelphia, USA: Mosby Elsevier.

Johnson, S. B., Park, H.S., Gross, C. P. & Yu, J. B. (2017). Use of Alternative Medicine for Cancer and Its Impact on Survival. *Journal of the National Cancer Institute*, 110(1), 121–124. doi: 10.1093/jcni/djx145. Published 10 August 2017; retrieved 16 March 2018.

Memorial Sloan Kettering Cancer Center. "Essiac." https://www.mskcc.org/cancer-care/integrative-medicine/herbs/essiac#references-5. Retrieved 04 Aug 2018.

Offit, Paul A. (2013). *Do You Believe in Magic? The sense and nonsense of alternative medicine*. USA: HarperCollins.

Richardson, M.A., Sanders, T., Palmer, J.L., Greisinger, A., Singletary, E. (2000). Complementary/Alternative Medicine Use in a Comprehensive Cancer Center and the Implications for Oncology. *Journal of Clinical Oncology*. doi: 10.1200/JCO.2000.18.13.2505

Russell, J. (Ed.) & Rovere, A. (Ed. Assistant) (2009). *American Cancer Society Complete Guide to Complementary and Alternative Cancer Therapies* (2nd ed.). Georgia, USA: American Cancer Society / Health Promotions.

Singh, Simon & Ernst, Edzard (2008). *Trick or Treatment? Alternative medicine on trial*. London, UK: Transworld Publishers.

Smith, J. A. (08 Sep 2015). Ten Questions to Ask about Scientific Studies. *Greater Good Magazine*. https://greatergood.berkeley.edu/article/item/10_questions _to_ask_about_scientific_studies

Turner, K. A. (2014). *Radical Remission: Surviving Cancer Against All Odds*. New York: HarperCollins Publishers.

RESOURCES:

Cochrane (*cochrane.org)*

National Cancer Institute (*cancer.gov*)

National Institutes of Health (*nih.gov*)

PubMed (*ncbi.nlm.nih.gov/pubmed/*)

Quackwatch (*quackwatch.org*)

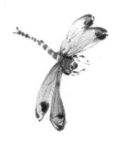

Chapter 18

A Transformational Journey
With and Through Cancer

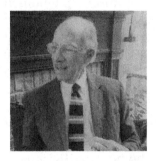

Alan S. Wolkenstein, MSW, ACSW

I was not diagnosed with anal cancer; however, I have lived through a diagnosis of prostate cancer, and I have been living with it for over 20 years now. People who are given a cancer diagnosis share many similarities. Anal cancer and prostate cancer affect similar areas in our bodies. My personal story, educational background, and work with other men and couples facing cancer is shared here to help others. I encourage you to take away some wisdom and tips on how to cope with your cancer diagnosis. I will share my cancer transformation journey, my reflections, the emotional components, how I helped others, and how relationships and sexuality are important topics to discuss. You will also hear my thoughts on the term "cancer survivor" and how I moved forward.

Alan S. Wolkenstein

The Whispering Voice Deep Within

A diagnosis of cancer and a grim prognosis can easily overwhelm all our senses, strip away our coping strategies, and destroy any semblance of a future. A diagnosis of cancer propels us, metaphorically, to the ends of the earth (Lifton & Olsen, 1974). The return back, for those of us able to attempt it, is a long and arduous journey. Having realized all this, I am writing about the personal transformation we experience by living with cancer. I believe such a transformation requires us to have experienced momentous loss and deep grieving.

It is this experience of the cancer losses and sustained lamentations/grieving-transformation phenomenon (or simply put, "cancer transformation process") that should be clarified if others are to understand our journey. To be fully engaged with us requires this awareness. I have lived with this threatening experience (prostate cancer), struggled and frequently failed to find a balance in my life, tried to stay focused on what is most important to my family and me, and repeatedly searched for the meaning of my life's experiences (Wolkenstein & Wolkenstein, 2009).

I remember returning home from the hospital. I ached; my body hurt; the stitches hurt. Nights were the worst, and I learned later from other men with prostate cancer they shared the unpleasantness of night-time as I did. The dreams were the most unpleasant. I ended up back in the hospital with a steady stream of visitors. They looked sad and worried, mostly. Most hugged me, but I was disconnected from my body, a cloud, eerily unpleasant in the room. I would wake up shaking.

Soon after, I heard a voice from deep within whispering for me to help myself, yet I did not understand how. The cancer had crept outside my prostate and was "incurable," so how could I help myself? To attempt to do so seemed like a cruel joke. My experiences and all I had learned until that time seemed to be of no assistance to me. I did not know how to cope or adapt to this, as never to be "me" again. Instead, I would be a person changed by my experiences and the events of my life. I tried not to lament the loss

176

of the old "me." Could I take these important challenges in stride as I struggled to look forward? I was desperately hoping there was a forward for me.

My Unique Perspective as a Fellow Traveler

We all have multiple inner voices that direct our thoughts and behaviors. We frequently require heightened awareness and a deeper understanding of these voices to more effectively lead us through the journey of life wherever it takes us.

I am a social worker and family therapist with a 30-year history of teaching behavioral sciences to resident physicians in Family Medicine and other primary care specialties. I am a man with a 20-year history of living with and through prostate cancer and a tough diagnosis. Additionally, soon after my diagnosis, I responded to a suggestion from my urologist to help others who are going through this type of cancer. He said I was the only therapist who could help because I was living it every day. I told him to have them call me. Soon these men referred their friends with the same diagnosis. As a result, as a fellow traveler, I have talked with over 100 men and their partners as a mentor and guide on their personal and extraordinary journey.

These three components of being a teacher, having lived through and with a cancer diagnosis, and helping others have provided me with a comprehensive and unique perspective.

My Experience Helping Others Affected by Cancer

I quickly found out talking with men and their families about prostate cancer was not about psychotherapy of any kind, but about mentoring, listening, and very, very cautious guiding. It was not about doing, but about being. Those of us in the helping professions seem ready to say and do but are impatient with simply being. The key, I found, for working with these men is about being there for them, "in the moment" (the Buddhist term is smriti) and not doing (Watts, 1960).

Meeting in cafes, restaurants, my car or theirs in their driveways, and often in their kitchens seemed better for conversations with me about who they were and where they were going. They talked about their feelings and thoughts seldom shared with others, even their family, friends, or physicians. Many were newly diagnosed or in various stages of healing. Others were barely living, just existing. I marveled at their desperate honesty. We were like an undercover club, a secret society of men, with the only membership requirement being a serious diagnosis like prostate cancer (Wolkenstein, Wolkenstein & Simona, 2004).

I learned how difficult it was to be a therapist when I shared the same illness. I struggled with the same issues. The men were satisfied with revealing experiences with someone who was ahead of them in their journey and genuinely able to validate their experiences and feelings as legitimate. That was fine with me. Their experiences and emotions were to be honored and explored, not diagnosed and treated; experiences and feelings accepted and not judged; experiences and feelings not assessed or evaluated. There were others to do that. I wanted to create a liminal experience with them, and for the most part, I have succeeded.

By liminal, I mean that cancer at first puts us in an ambiguous position. We suddenly have few, if any, certainties. The rules of life we knew are taken away, and we must begin the adaptation to a new world and life of healthcare specialists, health systems, hospitals, nurses, and physicians. Then to other people, our families, even our relationship with God. Nothing is the same, and few of us are skilled enough to make the adjustment alone. I learned that by being there for others, there was no need to be judgmental or critical. They needed this liminal experience to self-assess, self-learn, and realize the need to seek their deepest inner wisdom again (more on this later), regardless of whether they lost it as they lost their way in life, or dropped it because they believed it was of no value or it was too heavy to carry any farther. I emotionally walked alongside these men and worked to show them that somebody else was not afraid of the burdens they carried. I could accompany these people on their paths. We can benefit from mentors and guides who have been there and can light that pathway and suggest options we are unable to visualize.

Cancer is an Interpersonal Disease

The hormonal treatments sapped my strength and energy. I experienced physical and emotional changes, not in a regular progression as one ages, but at an unnatural and dizzying pace that forced me to confront again and again my identity as a man and to give up the expectations about what my body could and could not do.

I remember an incident during the first winter of remission of me walking up an icy hill in our yard from the garage. I carried a grocery bag in each arm, and the wind pushed into me from the front. I dropped the bags to keep from being blown down the hill and fell to one knee, cursing and crying out in shame and rage. An incline I had walked up a million times. Groceries I had carried for years without a problem. Could I ever return to any sort of normal life, and at the same time, pummel these losses, round after bloody round, until I could finally accept them, reframe them, and integrate them? At times, I could, and at other times I just could not.

As I grappled with this reality by myself and with my wife, Kathy, I became more aware of her losses, her fears, her worries about me and us. Would I live and who would I be? What would happen to us? What about our sons? She shared my loneliness, isolation, and fear, often silently. We then began to talk, really talk about us. We covered new ideas, and sometimes, old landscapes of unfinished issues from our past we both believed would be given plenty of "couple time" in the future to deal with and resolve. We realized we needed this "now time" to talk, not some far-off date in the future. Many times, I borrowed her strength to do this, and I am so appreciative of her. How did she keep her inner wisdom when I had discarded or maybe just lost mine? Other men also describe this realization that a partner who retains this deepest inner wisdom becomes a source of great strength, mentally, and even spiritually, for us.

Yes, there were times when this cancer would tap at the walls of my very being. It did not create the weaknesses and breaks and chips it found; it merely took advantage of them when it could. It seemed to look for weak spots in my marriage and me. Kathy and I learned, again and again, that cancer is an interpersonal disease and can conquer us if we lack healthy relationships and healthy support systems. Cancer affects our interpersonal lives, our deepest relationships, and our most intense interactions with important others and the world itself.

What has evolved for me over these decades? The assurance that Kathy and our sons Haran and Matthew always set a place for me in their lives.

The Reality of the Impermanence of Life

All of us, our partners and families, and sometimes even our physicians, are confronted by "impermanence." The reality is that we are born, we live, we die. On any level, it seems to make sense, but when stricken with cancer, the supports we used to live our lives in spite of knowing we will die one day are taken away. Suddenly, when cancer knocks us to our knees, the impermanence of life takes on an "in your face" reality. We have always lived with it, but now must accept, fully, if we are to truly cope with this cancer. Who are we? Where do we come from? Where are we going? Will we live or will we die? What are the new rules? Do we experience a rapidly changing relationship with God if we believe in God?

All bets are off for us. Our loved ones may see us afraid, outwardly and for the first time. Consider again that journey we have taken. The signposts for some are difficult to read, encoded, and shrouded in darkness. We may have a sense of hopelessness and helplessness. "If this is how we define a man (or woman), I would prefer to die. Maybe I should just let go—die and get it over with." For others, there is brightness and clarity. Why is it this way for some and not for others?

Over the years I have come to believe, from having so many conversations, that acceptance of impermanence may be a major key to successful coping. The way to an upright position after being knocked down, is to accept that we may die but to choose life. Accepting impermanence in life is not about giving up hope or faith in a future in which we are a part (Wolkenstein & Wolkenstein, 2008). To choose to live with and through cancer gives us a unique pathway we have created, even though the cancer was not of our choosing.

The Loss of Inner Wisdom

One other significant loss we may incur along with our physical and emotional ones is the loss of our deepest inner wisdom: a wondrous gift made up of our experiences, reflections and what we learned from them, and our beliefs, dreams, and wishes. It differs as to how aware we are of this gift of wisdom and our ability to use it in how we live our lives.

We lose it because we discard it in anger and sadness, believing it is no longer useful to us. Somehow it let us down before we became ill, and it weighs too much for us to carry on our journey. For me, it was important to reach out for it again. It did not let me down: I chose to believe it failed me and no longer had any purpose. This is just not so.

Let Us Talk About Sexuality

Whenever and wherever cancer strikes, we are overwhelmed with a dramatic change, fear, and the anxiety of the potential loss of our lives. No wonder we can become distant and feel disconnected from others, even with those we love and who love us. We tend to shy away from intimacy, mentally and physically, as if by being intimate we somehow open ourselves to further emotional pain and loss, pain and loss we cannot take on as additional burdens to our illness. Others reach out to us, but we frequently feel unable or even unwilling to respond positively. Our feelings are just too great and overwhelming.

Cancer of the prostate, breast, and anal canal are only but a few of the diseases that affect us in deeply personal places in our bodies. Places we perceived as private and personal are now exposed to physicians, nurses, and healthcare guides, generally in private physician offices or hospital settings. We are quickly educated by all these professionals to lose our inhibitions, for physical care involves them in direct and open ways. We lose our shyness; it is no wonder the drive for intimacy is weakened.

We may no longer feel sexy or desirable. Treatment robs us of both the desire and energy to be sexual. The losses of drive, desire, intimacy, and closeness are frequent by-products of treatment and medications. In addition, we have new worries, fears, and anxieties that cripple our basic human components of desire, interest, enthusiasm, and deeply felt physical and emotional intimacy. Will they return? It depends. Sometimes they return on their own with changes or elimination of some treatment and medication, sometimes by the passage of time as we attempt to rebalance our lives, and sometimes with the guidance of counselors and therapists skilled in the dynamics of living with and through cancer.

Any meaningful discussion of sexuality, whether or not we struggle with cancer, can create feelings of discomfort and anxiety among people. I believe those who have been diagnosed with and treated for prostate cancer (or other cancers affecting our private and personal parts) require such conversations, for they are extremely important and relevant for the person and his/her partner. I sense that people with extreme discomfort and anxiety may be dealing with experiences in their family of origin in which discussions of sex were not acceptable or appropriate. As adults, many people are still not able to permit themselves to have meaningful conversations about their sexuality.

Prostate cancer and other pelvic-area cancers and their treatments can all contribute to difficulties in a couple's sexual satisfaction. Issues such as generalized anxiety, performance anxiety, body-changes anxiety, lower levels of interest, and fatigue/ stress/focus on multiple losses and lamentation (suffering), incontinence, difficulty getting and maintaining an erection, vaginal stenosis and/or pain—all can cause mild to severe couple sexual dissatisfaction.

Because most of our sexual behavior is learned, new pathways to sexual behavior and attitudes for couples can also be successfully learned. The model of "Non Demand-Non Sexual Pleasuring" is very helpful (Kaplan, 1974; Wedding & Stuber, 2010). A key is to return to the attitude that the purpose of sex is to have fun and relax. A couple must adopt this belief before they can be helped to seek again that earlier exploratory phase in their relationship in which they tested out ideas and behaviors in getting to know each other sexually. Since most treatments interfere in previous sexual practices, this is the time to renew the search for relaxation and pleasure under a new system of sexual enlightenment. To seek that elusive erection for him, an emphasis on penetrating her, or orgasm for either is a guaranteed failed experience for couples.

What I have come to know is couples need to learn how to value the intimate actions they had long since taken for granted. Couples are encouraged to return to touch, non-genital caressing, holding, dancing, massaging each other, the renewal of romance by saying "I love you," and all behaviors that are emotionally, physically, and spiritually rewarding in and of themselves. They describe so much of their lives as being out of their control; these behaviors are within their control and also strengthen a couple's mastery over their relationship. This is undeniably an incredibly important realization for them.

Taking Issue with the Term "Cancer Survivor"

Before I was diagnosed with prostate cancer, I never really liked the term "cancer survivor." After five years in remission from prostate cancer, I liked it even less when I would be referred to as a "cancer survivor." After twenty years in remission, I abhor it. It is my belief to be identified as a cancer survivor carries for me, and maybe others, just too much of a sense of being controlled by cancer, always to be defined as a survivor first and not as an individual, and a constant negative vibe.

The National Cancer Institute (*cancer.gov*) uses the term and means well, but I disagree. Their definition states, "A cancer survivor is one who remains alive and continues to function during and after overcoming a serious hardship or life-threatening disease. In cancer, a person is considered to be a survivor from the time of diagnosis until the end of life."

CONSIDER: The generic term "survivor" is used to describe a person who has lived through a brush with death. Serious illnesses and other harrowing experiences can put people in line with the loss of their lives. The word survivor comes from the French word "vive" meaning long live. It now loosely defines the experience of living through an event or situation that is touched with death. However,

I continue to believe the term is insufficient, for it does not examine the permanent imprint and resulting transformation on each person and the family it touches.

One does not live through any such experience of cancer without transformation, and I believe all transformation requires loss. An understanding and awareness of this cancer transformation process benefits not only ourselves but also those who support and guide us. I have lived with and through a life-altering and life-threatening cancer experience. I do not wish to be known as a cancer survivor, but as a man who struggled, and sometimes failed, in seeking balance in my life, trying to stay focused on what is most important, and searching for meaning in my life's experiences. These experiences transcend the term cancer survivor.

I don't like the term cancer survivor as this puts cancer first. Cancer should never go first because that is what our spirit hears from us, and that isn't healing. If I must, I prefer to use the term "survivor of cancer." I, survivor, first. Cancer, second. I don't want my spirit-body-emotions inhibited or owned by the word cancer. And survivors are thrivers, but that is another book.

Balancing, Focusing, Making Sense

We may yet be stronger than we think. "It never fails to amaze me what people are able to survive" (Ellis, 2004).

Survival is complicated and requires input from several sources we seldom think about: family, partners, friends, community caregivers, social organizations, non-professional or informal support persons, and healthcare professionals. However, we are severely hampered by the multitude of changes cancer brings that affect us with no real respite, no time to think about and reflect on them with our partners, no expansiveness of time to adjust. Losses are shouldered one upon the other. How we look at ourselves as men and women, how we define our masculinity and femininity, the changes in our bodies and an unpredictable world are as fearful to us as our innermost feelings. The grieving may be outwardly intense as it was for me, or inward, and never to be spoken of or shared.

I suggest to help us survive we need the following:

- ✓ Balancing: We need time to bring our world back into balance.

- ✓ Focusing: We need to be mindful of the task to bring our energies to bear on what is most important.

- ✓ Making Sense: We need to make sense of these experiences. We are all struggling to cope with a new world, new rules, new meanings, new realistic fears and concerns, and new alliances in a healthcare system that for many of us is confusing, impersonal, and frightening.

Three Uninvited Guests Including the Unheralded "It"

While our attempt to seek balance, focus, and meaning in our lives has affective or emotional components to it, many of us are understandably profoundly troubled by three intense feelings, which I call the "three uninvited guests." The first two are isolation and loneliness. How sad that the first emotional responses we create for ourselves are to feel isolated and alone, even when family and friends are there to support and love us.

Many men described feelings of disassociation from themselves and their partners, feeling they were drifting, alone and isolated, even when there were other people in the room. Pleas by our partners and family and friends to let them into our world seem pointless. We lack the skills to allow them in, at least at that moment. While I played this important scenario out in dreams, other men would speak of it with me.

Sometimes, and not always, my clients will share with me their experiences with "it"—the third uninvited guest. "It" appeared to me as well. "It" comes unannounced, unheralded, in the middle of the night, without warning and fanfare. "It" wraps itself around our insides and squeezes until we cannot catch a breath as we recoil from its terrifying intensity. If we are asleep, "it" wakes us up. "It" is fear. We have told no one, shared this with no one. Not our partners, not our families, and certainly not our physicians. We may say to ourselves things like, "Alan, this is not something to share. What will others think? How can I tell my wife; she is so overburdened already? I am embarrassed by my weaknesses."

We already know such intense fears weaken our already compromised strength. "It" deflects us from trying to seek balance, to focus on what is most important, and to make sense out of what is happening to us (Wolkenstein & Wolkenstein, 2009).

We wait to see if "it" reappears. We wait and wait, and "it" doesn't. But then "it" may, however, in a modified and less intense way when we have tests or procedures, or assume the patient role in our healthcare system. Over time, "it" is diminished and presents as a less obstructive state. "This may sound strange, but I am not afraid of my fear anymore. Fear is something I can live with now. 'It' doesn't wake me anymore." In the place of fear, there may be quiet and stillness. For some of us, this may be the first time we are truly still within our thoughts and ourselves.

How I Moved Forward

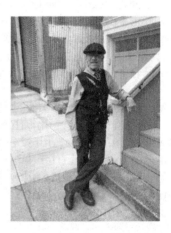

In order for me to move forward, I believe it helped that I chose guided imagery, meditation, affirmation, tai chi, biking, jazz, gentle conversations with our rabbi (that helped return me to my faith), periodic psychotherapy, prayer and contemplation alone and with my faith-based group, nutritional supplements, dietary assistance, and especially long walks filled with conversation with my wife Kathy.

I learned that each activity served and still serves as an essential posture in my healing:

- To boost my immune system.

- To reduce the sense of feeling lost and increase my self-understanding so I could more consciously choose my path of living. Now I know what Thoreau meant when he said, "It is not until we are lost that we begin to understand ourselves."

- To work to always be present by appreciating all our experiences while we are engaged in them. Now I understand what our son Matthew pointed out early on, "Dad, savor all moments with the ones you love."

- To not forget your partner's needs. Remembering he/she mourns all the same losses you do and may be overlooked during times of crisis and stress. Consider asking what is needed from you. It is as stressful for your significant other as for you.

- There may be times you have to let go of what is happening to you. It would seem counterintuitive to do so, especially when we feel so out of control and victimized by our circumstances. As it was for me, the more I let go, the more in control I was of those things I could realistically affect. I could control what I thought and felt if I let myself believe so. With such power, I could make a future for myself and my partner with me in that shared future. For many of the men I saw, I needed to go over this concept many times since it seemed so wrong to them. I learned the old adage that sometimes we do not understand what we choose not to understand. It is a model of great importance for and a challenge to share with men.

- To live our lives with purpose and meaning, even while we are in dire straits. This is about having a mission for our existence. Reflect on what your mission is. For many, it is doing what we love for as long as we can.

- I encouraged each man with whom I talked to find his own personal means and strategies to assist him and his family.

- I discovered that mentoring other men strengthened my resolve and energy.

Transformation Is Ongoing

If we regain our deepest personal wisdom, if we strive to return from the ends of the earth, if we see those critical signposts with clarity and brightness, if others continue to make a place for us in their lives, then our transformation is ongoing.

When we have endured the diagnosis and treatments of cancer, mourned our losses, and found the strength to carry on—then and only then will we be transformed. We are the same person, but different; we are fundamentally moved emotionally and spiritually by our experiences. We are taking a journey that was not our choice, but on a path we have chosen for ourselves, and we have a perspective unique to us as individuals.

There is frequently an enormity of sorrow that must be skillfully addressed if we are to grow to our personal (and sometimes couple) potential as part of our transformation (Muller, 1992). This requires us to live with and through cancer as an interpersonal disease not be lived with alone or experienced alone. It is not a personal disease, or a relationship disease, or even a family disease. It is interpersonal because it affects us personally in our relationships and in our families. While it may not appear relevant in a theoretical model to view it this way, it affects how we use our energy in our daily lives and interactions.

If we cannot allow ourselves to view this cancer as interpersonal, we will become frozen in time. If we cannot live with this cancer as interpersonal, we will "rigidify" our experiences to where living is all or nothing, black or white. We will minimize life without the real-time complexities that are there for us to enjoy and to be part of. All of this requires self-awareness, a skill lacking in some people, especially men. Can it be learned? Yes, with proper mentoring and guidance.

"When that inevitable moment comes, often in crisis, it can change our lives forever. We can no longer live our lives by accident. It breaks us open so that we watch our lives with excruciating care and we walk on the earth paying infinitely close attention to what is precious and what is true and what is right" (Muller, 1997).

An earlier version of this paper was published in 2009 online: myprostatecancerroadmap.com.

****

REFERENCES:

Ellis, Mary (2004). *The Turtle Warrior*. New York: Viking Press.

Kaplan, Helen Singer (1974). *The New Sex Therapy*. New York: Brfunnerand Mazel.

Lifton, R. and Olsen E. (1974). *Living and Dying*. New York: Prager.

Muller, Wayne (1992). *Legacy of the Heart: The Spiritual Advantage of a Painful Childhood*. New York: Simon and Schuster.

National Cancer Institute (NCI) Dictionary of Cancer Terms. https://www.cancer.gov/publications/dictionaries/cancer-terms

Watts, Alan (1960). *This is It and Other Essays on Zen and Spiritual Experience*. New York: Vantage Books.

Wedding, D. and Stuber, M. (Eds.) (2010). *Behavior and Medicine*. Gogttingen Germany: Hogreteand Huber.

Wolkenstein, Alan S., Wolkenstein, M. Evan, and Simona, K. (2004). The Card: An Educator's Encounter With Cancer. *Family Medicine*, 36(2); 137-140.

Wolkenstein, Alan S. and Wolkenstein, M. Evan (2008). The Continuing Journey: A Guide to the Cancer Experience. *Annals of Behavioral Science and Medical Education*, 14(2); 85-86.

Wolkenstein, Alan S. & Wolkenstein, M. Evan (January/February, 2009). Signposts of the Cancer Journey. *Coping Magazine*.

Wolkenstein, Alan S. and Wolkenstein, M. Evan (2009). Using Reflective Learning in Medical Education and Practice. *Medical Encounter.* 23(3); 97-102.

Additional Resources:

Annon, J. (1976). *Behavioral Treatment of Sexual Problems.* New York: Harper and Row.

Frankl, Viktor (1998). *The Will to Meaning: Foundations and Applications of Logotherapy.* New York: Penguin Books.

Friedman, H. (1992). *The Self-Healing Personality: Why Some People Achieve Health and Others Succumb to Illness.* New York: Penguin Books.

Muller, Wayne. *Touching the Divine.* Audio Books, 1997.

Lastly, here are two papers that lend additional information specific to men, anal cancer and sexuality:

Men's Guide to Sexuality During and After Cancer Treatment (OncoLink, 2017): https://www.oncolink.org/support/sexuality-fertility/sexuality/men-s-guide-to-sexuality-during-after-cancer-treatment

Cancer Can Affect a Man's Desire and Sexual Response (American Cancer Society, 2017): https://www.cancer.org/treatment/treatments-and-side-effects/physical-side-effects/fertility-and-sexual-side-effects/sexuality-for-men-with-cancer/treatment-and-desire-and-response.html

Chapter 19

Cancer Blessings

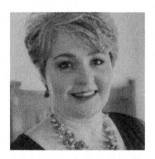

Peggy Belton

"Every experience, no matter how bad it seems, holds within it a blessing of some kind. The goal is to find it." –Buddha

It seems like just yesterday. A lump. I knew it was cancer. Even worse, I knew I was going to die just like Farrah Fawcett. My heart raced and panic pulsed through my veins. "Help!"

I came out of the bathroom with tears streaming down my face and blurted it out, "I have a lump in my butt, and I am going to die like Farrah Fawcett." My husband thought I was crazy. "What? Slow down. You're not going to die." He tried to convince me that I was overreacting and that once I saw a doctor, everything would be fine. It was that moment I knew my life had just changed—I thought for the worse.

Three days later, my medical journey began with a routine Pap smear, which quickly became an invasive rectal exam. I'd never been happier to have someone want to stick a finger up my rump. While anal cancer was on the list of differentials, since it was a gynecologist doing the poking, invasive endometriosis was a potential diagnosis as well. Oh, how I wanted to believe that could be true, but my gut knew better. I was scheduled for a colonoscopy a couple of weeks later.

The Lurking Lump

Incidental to everything going on down yonder, I had a whole body mole check done, and the Physician Assistant removed six moles and sent them to pathology to rule out melanoma. I wasn't worried in the least. I've been down that road before, and the biopsies always came back normal, at least they did before. My mind couldn't stop thinking about how hard the lump was in my butt. I became obsessed with Googling images of anal cancers and hemorrhoids, trying to compare my lump as I imagined it with the ones on the Internet. Even when I was driving down the highway, I was looking on my phone at images of anal cancer and reading articles about the human papillomavirus (HPV) and squamous cell carcinoma.

I tried to go on with my life as always, attempting to distract myself with my work. Emails, reports, site visits, meetings with hospital executives, and spending time supporting my direct reports and their staff should have been enough to keep any mind busy, but the thought of the lump was always lurking. I recall one day in particular, I was working with one of my employees, a Program Director. We were out in the community meeting with physicians. As always when I work away from my home office, my phone was set to silent. We got back to her car and decided it was time for lunch. As we headed over to Subway, I noticed I had missed a call. I remember that Dermatology Physician Assistant (PA) telling me, "If everything is normal, we will send you a card in the mail. Otherwise, we will call you."

Seriously? I don't need this now; I have a lump in my butt! I can't deal with two cancers.

The First Cancer Diagnosis

Of course, it had to be lunch hour when I tried to return the call to Dermatology. When I finally got through, the nurse told me that I needed to come in to get my results. I left my Program Director and drove back to town as fast as I could to meet my husband, who was waiting at the office when I got there.

We got the news that we had dreaded—it was melanoma, and I was going to need minor surgery to remove a large area of tissue. The news of the melanoma made my anxiety shoot through the roof so, of course, I Googled. What a mistake! When you Google melanoma and rectal mass in the same search, you find out you're going to die. At this point, I had four more days left until my colonoscopy.

The colonoscopy day finally arrived, and I was so happy that I might get an answer to what was going on in my hind end. I couldn't wait to see the pictures. They always take pictures. I told my husband, "Make sure Doc gives you the pictures." I told the nurses, "Please make sure he takes pictures. I need to see the pictures." Everyone knew I was desperate to see what the heck was growing inside of me. Then the drugs kicked in, and for what seemed like a moment, my mind was quiet.

The Second Cancer Diagnosis

As I came to, I opened my eyes to find my husband waiting with me. The nurse told me I could get dressed, and moments later, the doctor came in with my pictures. I was immediately alert. He went on to point out the mass I felt and said he was concerned it was cancer. He also pointed out the picture of a huge mass that was almost completely blocking my rectum, which he could not speculate as to what it was. The next three days would be the longest days of my life.

The call came. I had squamous cell carcinoma that was most likely a result of having HPV, and an obstructing mass that must have been growing on the outside of my rectum because the biopsy for that came back normal. I hung up the phone and told my husband the news, then immediately Googled. The first thing I read listed an overall survival rate of 38%. I cried.

My husband and I went for a drive, and both sobbed our eyes out. I was going to die. I wasn't ever going to be a grandma. I wasn't ready to die! My husband! My kids! This was my fault because I have HPV as a result of unprotected sex. Everyone was going to think I had anal cancer because of anal sex. I felt so stupid, so dirty, and so ashamed! This couldn't be happening! But it was.

The Blessings Begin

Rewind about a week, Saturday night. We were at church, newly diagnosed with melanoma and listening to the sermon. We were trying to be calm, have faith, and trust in the Lord, but we were so afraid. After the service was over, we went up front to meet with one of the pastors or chaplains. That is when the blessings began, even though it would take me another week to realize it.

Pastor Chip was happy to see us. I fought through the tears and embarrassment to open up to him and share the details of the melanoma and the lump in my butt. I will never forget his words, "Pay attention to not only what He is doing in you, but what He is doing through you." Chip's prayer changed my world!

Within a few short days of receiving the anal cancer diagnosis, my focus began to shift. I was still anxious about the treatment I would have to go through, but I found myself looking outward, thinking about how I could become a servant to others through this journey. I realized my struggle could help someone else and began blogging. I was determined to be honest, brutally honest, in my blogs so others might learn about the risks of HPV, the need to vaccinate their children, and that anyone can get HPV and HPV-related cancer.

My cancer treatment began about a month after receiving the diagnosis, but the blessings started appearing almost immediately. The first thing I realized was God had spoken to me four months earlier during my company's benefit enrollment period. My husband and I had been married for two years. We both had health insurance through our employers, but this year, I found myself contemplating the need to add myself to my husband's policy to have secondary coverage. My husband, Guy, added me to his plan, and four months later, we were thanking God for that nudge as it meant cancer would not become a financial burden to our family. By the end of that year, our insurance had been charged more than $300,000 USD, but as a result of acting on the spiritual nudge and having that secondary insurance, my care cost us less than $4,000 USD.

The next blessing came in the form of clinical care and medical expertise. I was blessed with a referral to the Mayo Clinic for further diagnostics and treatment planning. The nurses and physicians were top-notch. In addition to being well-versed on the cancer I had, the many physicians involved in my case were caring, compassionate, and readily available. They worked as a team. Not the kind of medical team who works together by sending you to a different office every few days or weeks, communicating through transcribed progress notes, but the type of team that actually huddles and discusses cases together. They collaboratively reviewed my test results and developed a treatment plan.

My medical oncologist, the chemo doctor, was so kind and gentle. She and her team of infusion nurses made sure I understood my treatment and were fantastic about addressing any unpleasant side effects to the best of their ability. Whenever I would express my misery, they were quick to reassure me that I was not creating a burden to them, and they were pleased to help.

The radiation oncologist was also wonderful. While he had a very serious demeanor, his resident physician spent a considerable amount of time educating me and making all the arrangements for my care. They wanted me to do my treatments at their facility so they could give me what they believed was superior care. I expressed concern about lodging since I lived 2.5 hours away. The resident physician made a referral for me to the Hope Lodge, a hotel-like facility affiliated with The American Cancer Society, which provides free lodging for patients receiving radiation therapy. Even with 65 guestrooms, there was a three-week waiting list, and I was on it.

I started my six weeks of treatment by staying at a hotel across from the clinic. It was mediocre, but since I slept most of the time, it was sufficient. The morning of the fifth day, my youngest daughter, who had been coordinating vet care for our ailing Feline Leukemia-positive cat, called to tell us that Mr. Whampus' health had deteriorated to the point of needing to be put down. Again, we cried. It seemed so unfair while dealing with cancer we would lose our beautiful Maine Coon boy. A few moments later, we received another call. This time it was the Hope Lodge informing me a room had opened up for me two weeks ahead of schedule—another blessing that would save us thousands of dollars.

God's blessings aren't always so obvious. Sometimes they don't happen to you but through you. I believe God worked through me in many ways. While I don't believe God gave me cancer, I do believe He used that opportunity to work through me for my benefit as well as others around me.

The Most Profound Blessing

One of the most profound blessings was witnessing the impact my cancer had on my daughters. In the beginning, I think they were in shock, which turned into fear, but they tried to hide their concerns and remain positive. As my treatment journey progressed and my discomfort got worse, I watched them both become protectors and caregivers. In a matter of a few weeks, they both matured tremendously.

My oldest daughter became the most compassionate, attentive caregiver I could have imagined. It was the last day of treatment, and the burns on my bottom coupled with diarrhea from the chemo were causing terrible pain. The only way I could clean up was to get in the shower and use the hand sprayer to rinse myself off. I was so weak, and the pain was so great, I dropped to my knees and sobbed. As I lay on the shower floor, I began passing more stool uncontrollably. It was at that moment I got to see how my cancer had turned my child into a woman. She got down on her knees and began to push the mess away from me, so I didn't have to lie in my own feces. She never hesitated or curled her nose but did what needed to be done. I was so helpless, so weak, and so proud.

My youngest daughter didn't hesitate to step up and become my caregiver either. When I finally got to come home for good, I was physically at my worst. The radiation burns were excruciatingly painful and required topical medications and dressings that had to be changed every time I went to the bathroom. Can you imagine being 21 years old having to get up close and personal with your mother's hoo-ha and butthole? Again, I was a proud mama seeing her care for me without expressing any displeasure whatsoever. All she wanted to do was help me feel better.

Those girls became women, women who love their mother, and their mother was blessed.

Deepening Faith

I mentioned previously, I started blogging about my journey. I shared what I was going through and how my faith was getting me through it. I posted my blog on my Facebook page and received many comments and well wishes. It felt good, but when I returned to work, I was surprised by the number of people who shared their stories of faith with me. Several people expressed experiencing my journey through my words deepened their own faith in God. One business colleague even referred to me as his "answered prayer."

Advocating for HPV Vaccine

The blog and Facebook were where I first began to advocate for HPV vaccination. On a personal level, I was always an advocate for the HPV vaccines. Having had cervical cancer at the age of 22, I asked our pediatrician to give my girls the Gardasil vaccine before it was even available for purchase. It seemed like a "no-brainer." I am so glad because of my decision to vaccinate my daughters, they should never have to go through the misery that so many others and I have endured because of the human papillomavirus.

Becoming more of an advocate would mean I would have to shed the shame I had carried as an HPV-positive woman for years. If I was going to influence anyone to take steps to protect their children, I was going to have to get comfortable talking about HPV and my experience. So, I prayed for courage, and He blessed me with courage. Now when I talk to others about my cancer, I make sure to share that HPV indeed caused my cancer, and there is a vaccine that can prevent others from having to know what anal cancer feels like.

At this point in my journey, almost a year since my diagnosis, I am just scratching the advocacy surface. I have hopes of working with community groups and media outlets to share my story and motivate parents to protect their children from a painful future through vaccination.

Continuing to Feel Blessed After Treatment

It's been eight months since my cancer treatment ended. The skin has healed. The primary tumor has disappeared. The baseball-sized mass continues to shrink, and the other lymph nodes are reducing in size too. The doctors say there is no evidence of active disease. I am blessed!

Life isn't perfect or normal like it used to be. I have a quite a few side effects from the radiation that I will most likely have to live with for the rest of my life. Some people would become depressed by these changes, and some might have changes so significant that they might not be able to work, but again I am blessed. Blessed because my side effects remind me that I am ALIVE!

Don't get me wrong. I can throw myself a pity party from time to time, but living with hip pain and stiffness, some leg swelling, and a vagina that is trying to close are all worth it to be able to have more time on Earth. I am reminded on a daily basis I have a new normal. Every time I go to the bathroom, I am aware I am surviving what could have been a death sentence. What a blessing! Not to mention that through my relationship with Christ, I have developed a sense of peace with the side effects and physical limitations.

As a "can-do" kind of gal, I have always been a take-charge, self-sufficient problem solver. While having that personality type may have gotten me a high-level leadership position at work, it also got me a lot of gray hair, sleepless nights, and countless hours of mental anguish. Having to deal with the effects of radiation on a daily basis has caused me to accept my physical limits and realize that I do not need to be self-sufficient—I can humble myself and graciously accept help from others. How blessed am I to have this breakthrough before it's too late?

He is in Control

The word "cancer" invokes strong emotions in almost everyone I know, except perhaps my oncologists. Fear, sorrow, insecurity, or even anger wash over the person with cancer as well as their family, friends, co-workers, and even acquaintances. Often, we go into "fix-it" mode: trying to fix the situation, cheering up the person diagnosed with cancer, and supporting those around us. It's almost human nature to feel responsible for finding a way to handle what is placed before us. It was certainly how I responded in the past.

I, like many Christians, struggle to accept that I am not in control, He is. This cancer journey has helped me to trust in Him, to relinquish my need to control. Talk about peace!

> But blessed is the one who trusts in the Lord,
> whose confidence is in Him.
> They will be like a tree planted by the water
> that sends out its roots by the stream.
> It does not fear when heat comes;
> its leaves are always green.
> It has no worries in a year of drought
> and never fails to bear fruit.
> —Jeremiah 17:7-8 NIV

There is something so freeing about leaning into the Lord in times of stress. When we feel like we have to find the solution, the answer, the compromise, we bear the burden. He doesn't want us to bear those burdens, but our faith is often not strong enough to trust in Him completely.

> Trust in the Lord with all your heart
> and lean not on your own understanding;
> in all your ways submit to Him,
> and He will make your paths straight.
> —Proverbs 3:5-6 NIV

Handing My Struggles Over to Him

For me, I must admit, I struggled for a bit, and then I prayed about it and made the conscious decision to hand my struggles over to

Him. Once I decided to lean into Him, my anguish began to diminish. Instead of occupying my mind with uncertainty and fear, I was able to focus all of my energy on my treatment and doing what I needed to do to get through those physically challenging weeks. When I would feel weak, I would remind myself of one of my favorite scriptures:

> I can do all this through him who gives me strength.
> –Philippians 4:13 NIV

It was a great reminder that He was giving me the strength I needed, and if something was meant to be, He would provide what is required. I am blessed!

It would be easy for me to wallow in grief and self-pity as a cancer patient. I could focus on the fact that my cancer was a stage 3B, which means that in addition to the primary tumor, the cancer has metastasized to lymph nodes beyond the immediately adjacent area known as the perirectal area. According to the American Cancer Society, the five-year survival rate for stage 3B anal cancer is 43%– not exactly the most promising statistic.

Focus on the Blessings Instead of the Negatives

I could focus on the fact the cancer treatment destroyed my sex life. Radiation causes significant amounts of inflammation and burning, and scar tissue forms during the healing process. The scar tissue tries to adhere to itself and makes the vagina narrow and less flexible. It is hard to enjoy being intimate with your spouse when the experience feels like having sex with a knife! At the ages of 47 and 54, my husband and I are not ready to stop making love.

I could focus on the hip pain and stiffness, the fact that I can't lie on my side in bed without my top hip feeling like I did some serious weight lifting the day before. Or that those stiff hips make it hard to spread my legs apart or squat down to pick something up. When I stand up after sitting for a while, my hips function like my mother's hips who is 24 years my senior with a history of a previous hip fracture.

I could focus on how miserable my life has become due to the hot flashes induced by the radiation therapy. Ok, I have to confess . . . those hot flashes are hard to ignore. Essentially, the radiation fried my ovaries and put me into early menopause, which triggered the hot flashes. I am sure being overweight doesn't help the discomfort that goes along with them. I've also been told caffeine and alcohol can exacerbate hot flashes, but a girl needs her "pick me up" and "chill me out" vices, so I'm going to have to find another way to work through this issue.

I could keep going on about the negatives, but where would that get me? Right where I don't want to be–stressed out! My point? Happiness is a CHOICE! By focusing on the blessings that the good Lord afforded me through this cancer journey, I have landed in a good place. My marriage is stronger, my relationship with my daughters has deepened, my faith is part of every day, people share with me the impact I make on their lives, and I know now more than ever how much I am loved. I am blessed!

I know my life's path is still uncertain. Who really knows what the future holds? This cancer has blessed me with the opportunity to focus on the right things, the important things, today. I can stop stressing out by not trying to control everything and trust in what Christ is doing in and through me. I have received the opportunity to do all of this before it is too late. I've been given the blessing of time and awareness. I know it shouldn't have taken anal cancer to realize what is important, but it did, or at least it took getting cancer to realize I had to align my actions with my priorities.

Nevertheless I am continually with You;
You have taken hold of my right hand.
With Your counsel You will guide me,
And afterward receive me to glory.
–Psalm 73:23-24

Chapter 20

The Power of a Mother's Love

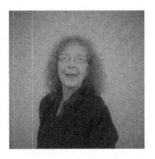

Virginia Davis Wilson

My chaotic life had finally leveled off after years of losses, struggling, and trying to reboot into the normal, manageable swing of things. This was March 2017. Then, unexpectedly, the heart-piercing phone message from my daughter Angela came. I will always remember it as it is deeply tattooed in my "Mother-Love" memory bank.

"Mom, I have a lump in my rectum. I will be undergoing a colonoscopy soon."

Initially, an ice-cold veil of horror, death, and end-of-the-world thinking fell over me. "No!" my psyche screamed. "I won't accept this. I am in charge of my thoughts." I then decided she had an abscessed hemorrhoid. "There! I like that! Treatable! Not life-threatening! There, done!" This held me for 24 hours. Almost obsessively, I had to find facts to hold on to, be they real or not. At this stage, it transformed into, "All about me."

The Strength and Power of Prayer

Angela was going for an urgent colonoscopy on April 13th. She emailed a prayer to me. I felt she had tapped into a power outside of herself. Angela wasn't succumbing to her affliction; she was going to fight the fight and look for strength and power to carry her through. It was comforting as we were feeling grave uncertainty at this time.

Dear Lord,

As my loved ones and I await the results of medical tests about my affliction, let us offer you our anxieties for our good and your glory. Calm us in our worries, knowing these don't add wisdom but rather stress to this situation. Enlighten us, through the power of your Spirit, to make wise decisions as to treatment. Help us not to turn away from You in these fragile, painful moments, but rather toward you for grace and strength. Comfort us in seeking you now, placing all our concerns in your loving hands as we say 'Thy Will Be Done.'

Amen

I Choose to Suffer Along

Many miles separate us, so Angela shared the results on the phone. "Mom, I have cancer, Stage 3 anal cancer." Sobbing saturated her words. "Oh, my darling! My perfect upstanding daughter! No! No! No!" reverberated in my brain. I was in disbelief. I feared not being able to handle this mentally or physically.

I instantly chose to become just as vulnerable to this diagnosis. I willingly wanted to suffer along, be there totally, heart and soul. I accepted this for myself. It vividly proved my unconditional, undying love for my daughter. I owed this penance to our relationship. What else could I do? This shock had taken me by such surprise, I needed a plan (for my own suffering in honor of my daughter), and this is it to the extreme.

Certain songs grabbed and jerked my attention constantly, such as, "Don't Leave Me This Way" by Thelma Houston and "Wind Beneath

My Wings" by Bette Midler. These songs fueled my thoughts and feelings of helplessness. Some songs emphasized the need I had to suffer along with her. Others motivated me to experience personal mental pain and distress in honor of her physical suffering. I made an oath unto myself: "I will die a compassionate death if something happens to Angela. She is my lifeline."

Arming Myself with Facts and Hope

I feverishly started studying up on all I could about cancer as never before via Google, TedTalks, and library books. My reading material fluctuated from medical facts to awesome healing powers and regimes. I developed an insatiable thirst for facts and cures to arm me against this mysterious, silent invader. I waited, wondering and studying statistics to no avail. Now I had become a "different" kind of victim of the "Big C." As alien as this fight would be, I was there for the long haul. I became so emotionally involved that I developed irritable bowel syndrome and suffered for months.

Four Friends Offer Four Messages of Hope

"Some people go to priests; others to poetry; I to my friends."
–Bernard, *The Waves*, Virginia Woolf

A self-proclaimed "diction-addict" (dictionary addict, my word), my nose is always in the Oxford Canadian Dictionary of Current English. I don't condemn myself. We are all looking for answers. Individually, personally, we all find our go-to sources. For me, I relied greatly on my friends. In my case, "friend" meaning, 1) a person with whom one enjoys mutual affection and regard, 2) a sympathizer, 3) an ally, sympathizer, or patron, 4) a romantic or sexual partner, 5) an acquaintance. Also, to be friends with is to be on good or intimate terms with.

I shall proceed with briefly sharing my experiences with four of my influential friends' input regarding my mental turmoil—"A state of great disturbance." They are all unique individuals. I like to call them divine messengers. I can feel God's power through our phone chats and face-to-face visits. I celebrate their friendships, enduring mutual life experiences together. We are there for each other, unconditionally and faithfully without abandonment. "Friends are people who help you be more yourself. More the person you were intended to be" (Merle Shain).

Joann—I confessed to Joann that I was "losing it" and wanted to give in to the craving for my own demise. To me, it was a proclamation of the depth of my mother-love. Sternly and supportively she chirped, "Oh, no, you need to be there for her and what she is going through." It brought me to my senses. I needed to be strong for my daughter.

Cathy—I let her know what my daughter was going through. At that point, I was in negative mode. She curtly said, "She'll be fine." Those words stayed with me because I value her friendship and all that she had been through.

Terri—When she called, I told her the situation. She offered prayers. Terri is a faithful church supporter. Life has been hard on her. Her faith in God carries her through day-by-day.

Barb—Over the phone, my long-distance friend offered words of hope and positive stories of people she knows who survived a cancer diagnosis.

My faith in the strength of friendships has changed dramatically for the better. Four styles, four friends, four inspirational pep talks. They are all so unique and nurturing. My floundering thoughts take it all in. They are like diamonds in the rough. The song "That's What Friends are For" by Dionne Warwick plays in my mind, confirming the reason why connections and friendships are so important.

Writing in My Journal

Writing in a journal is not at all foreign or an awkward activity for me. I would consider myself a five-star journaler. This time, however, I was in a shaky new state of mind. In this icy cold beginning and diagnosis, I felt alone, unarmed for what I was about to endure. Was I going to be powerless as a protective mother for my daughter newly diagnosed with cancer? What was going to be thrown at her and me? Yes. It immediately felt as if we were both suffering with anal cancer. Both of us were crumbling in shock. We were newbies at this. It was horrible mentally, physically and spiritually. I had no concrete thoughts toward coping or dealing with this life-threatening demon.

My first sense of who to lash out at was the elusive, invisible power of God. I had nowhere else to go at that point. As a Christian, my instinct in the face of cancer was, justifiably, to attack my Creator. Anything having to do with life and death is undoubtedly His responsibility, says I. My writing allowed me to safely and sincerely sort out my fear-driven thoughts. I even sensed having some power of control over my daughter's welfare.

As I wrote, more hate and fear bubbled up to the surface of my soul, then something clicked. A revelation popped into my thinking. Was this the power of God? This wasn't me! I needed to get a grip, or I would be useless to myself, my daughter, and our fighting journey we were about to face. *There is no hope or power in negative thinking*. Wow! What a sense of enlightenment. Who was speaking to me?

Frantically, I continued to read books, looking for scraps of knowledge. It served as an occasional slight comfort. Then I read Eckhart Tolle's book, *A New Earth*. The calming, focused answer for me was at the end of the book. He states to live fulfilled, we must experience acceptance, enjoyment, and enthusiasm. I changed enthusiasm to enlightenment in my personal notes because I could. Enthusiasm means intense and eager pleasure in an activity, an awakened purpose with a goal and a vision. I chose enlightenment, which means an understanding or awareness of something that brings change. I decided then and there I would become a positive, hopeful vessel for God's strength and power to work here on earth, enabling my daughter to be restored back to health.

Just changing my thinking opened up so much for me: mother-daughter love, faith in healing, trust in the medical system, and renewed powerful, awesome love of God. Answers, support, and healing are the theme of this journey, a beautiful thing.

Our Spiritual Strength Grew

Angela kept me close to her heart and emailed me prayers that are helpful to her in hopes it may also provide me with some comfort:

Dear Lord,

Please hold me close at this time of uncertainty.
Remind me of your promises when I am feeling overwhelmed.
Whisper words of love when I feel alone.
Lay me down in peace when I am weary.
Give all who care for me great waves of wisdom.
Lead me through this journey singing songs of hope over my life.
Quiet my soul as I face treatment of this anal cancer.
Come quell the fears I have, and fill my heart and mind with your everlasting love.
I will let you carry me when I feel weak or when I am suffering.
Thank you for my healing.

Amen

Being so far away, I felt my daughter is finding tangible answers in these spiritual prayers. I noticed her spiritual strength was growing and developing to comfort her. I felt as though it was a surrogate mother helping her because I was not right there.

I found a comforting prayer for myself from Andrew Weil's book *Spontaneous Healing*:

Dear Lord,

If you are my true God of love, power, and healing, please leave our angel here on earth as she has so much more love and work to share for the good of humanity. Make her life keep shining brightly, and her energy bring peace to all she encounters. I pray this in the name of the Father, Son, and Holy Ghost. Heal my daughter completely.

Amen

An Indelible Moment in Time

Angela called, wounded emotionally, sobbing, and wanting to vent to me. It was an honor, not defamation of her character. Honored that she knew her mother, where she was, and that I was alive and open to her needs. This was such an incredible bond, a beautiful moment—not every mother gets to share this experience with her child. Rich, real, warranted, and I was able to take it in. I buffered the emotional floundering for her. I was there, really there, and felt honored to be needed. This went way beyond everyday life. It was a soul-tugging and spiritual bonding. I will never forget it.

This vulnerable God-like moment of interaction was the apex to having given birth to my daughter. My tears as I write this verify such. What I'm trying to say is that super-human powerful moments are there to be shared between mother and child. Watch, wait, and be aware. Would I ever thank cancer? The big question for me is why can't we elevate our relationship without being influenced by the Big C? That will remain a mystery.

Prayer to Our Lady of Perpetual Help

Angela shared this prayer she used daily to help her get through her difficult days:

O Mother of Perpetual Help,

With greatest confidence I present myself to you.
I implore your help in the problems of my daily life.
Trials and sorrows often depress me; painful privations bring heartache into my life; often I meet the cross.
Have pity on me, compassionate Mother.
Take care of my needs, free me from my sufferings, or, if it be the will of God that I should suffer still longer, grant that I may endure all with love and patience.
Mother of Perpetual Help, I ask this in your love and power.

Amen

Being There for Her

Angela needed and wanted me to be there for three weeks while she endured the nauseating, draining chemo and radiation, so I went. It was so special to be able to be right there with her and beside her at the daily appointments. I can't imagine not being there. We rode the pain and fear together. I wanted to share the physical pain with her but I couldn't. She could vent to her family and me in a humbling, excruciating way. We all had no choice but to live it the best way we could: being raw, accepting, and loving.

Her room was dark, always filled with the calming essence of lavender essential oil. Many gifts and cards of hope and inspiration filled the room. It never felt like a sick room to me; it was a healing space. Special drinks, food, and music surrounded us. There was a strong feeling of divinity in the bedroom. My daughter told me she saw the image of Jesus beside her one time when the pain from the radiation was unbearable.

All of a sudden I became my own self-acclaimed deep soul philosopher, "sans degree." Being a protective mother, I was determined for my daughter's sake to discover answers and, of course, healing cures. In that frame of mind, I am always furthering my study course on cancer. I instructed her to stand up to this foe with all her personal tools of character and strength, whatever they may be. I reassured her that *she* isn't cancer. It wouldn't rob her of who she is inside, ever. I wouldn't let it. Mother Bear. Together we stepped into this forced awareness of her deep soul truth. It was powerful to talk, share, and plan our program on the road to healing. I already knew her style of character and how she had always coped with normal living. However, this was very jarring. We were going to delve deep into what would carry and empower her through this temporarily dark time. We began.

I knew my daughter is an organizer, just as every mother understands her child's character. So be it. Her journey involved putting all the negative emotions aside and attacking this foe with organization skills. It comforted us both to feel she hadn't lost her true self. She and I wouldn't let that happen! It took much thought, action, and might. We wouldn't play the game of "Hang in there," "Wait and see," "Who knows?" It wasn't going to demolish my daughter, as we knew spiritually it could, leaving the victim defenseless and wilted.

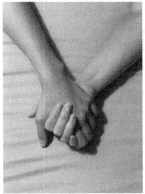

No doom and gloom! We held a positive mindset, knowing so much can be done nowadays to detect and cure cancer. It was an ugly program, and we were all helping to get to the healed end of it.

We both tapped into mutual special depths of consciousness and energy we never knew we had. We became vulnerable to each other's love and existence. That is how I describe it—very powerful in a positive direction. This mindset we developed as mother and daughter in the destructive face of cancer gave us an eternal bonding of power and hope. I felt with this arming of our inner souls, we would ride out the long, slow road ahead. This new attitude created incredible wisdom in us both.

Helping and Coping from Afar

Back home again, I reflected on what Angela was dealing with. My daughter organized her own focused, on-track procedures, which proved a blessing to me, being so far away. Her daily journal on the computer to select friends and family was something constantly watched for. We commented and read others' messages of strength and encouragement. It protected her from having to talk to us individually about her condition and progress. To me, she was the poster girl for how to trudge courageously through this cancer episode. Not a surprise—as she is a methodical, intense organizer. She kept us all in the loop as to what procedures, specialists, and outcomes were day by day.

This was so different from cancer in the 50s. I was told my grandmother had pancreatic cancer after she'd passed away. It was fast and a mystery. I heard after the fact that she could have had an operation, but Grampa felt it would spread faster if they opened her up. Things have come so far in sixty years. With modern day technology, it makes it easier to share, support and strengthen the loved one harboring cancer.

Defining Cancer

Back at home, thousands of miles away, while Angela waited for results of treatment, I decided to get out my trusty dictionary to try and define cancer. Why of all the human maladies did it have all this obnoxious power over the human body? Other diseases seem to follow a program or a script, which could be, to some degree of faith, watched and treated. Oh no, not cancer. It is the king of diseases. It is so powerful and in control of who, when, where it was going to hit and the amount of destruction it inflicts. I call cancer "empowered evil."

I started to wonder if an unexplainable cosmic-powered computer chip drives it. My distress had me clamoring for any slight upper-hand knowledge. Yes, it was getting to me! Back to the dictionary. I couldn't believe how many words starting with "ob" help define cancer. Obviate (get around), obscene, obnoxious, obscure, obtuse, oblivious, and obstinate. I am not kidding! Why did this give me a little comfort? I'll never know. I was digging for tangible answers, patterns, and causes. I had to let it go. It seemed to be enlarging the mystery of its phantom-like style.

Other diseases seem to play fair—signals, slow descent, a certain amount of preventative measures. Not cancer. It ambushes us, then hides until it's ready to expose itself on its own terms. Yes, I have a hate on for cancer. Who doesn't? Or wouldn't?

It took my best friend at 34, my grandmother at 67, my best friend's sister at 30, on and on it goes. No rhyme, no reason, or age limits.

Sending Words of Strength and Love

Angela informed me she was diagnosed with depression. She said it happens to many people who go through cancer treatment. I thought a lot about what she had gone through and emailed her this letter:

Dear Angela,

Part of your depression could be caused by the loss of your original ingrained self. Part of your healing involves reinventing yourself. Who you were before cancer served you well during that phase of your life. But now, your circumstances and priorities have forced you to change.

Reinventing ourselves is common and necessary as life rolls on. Life is full of change—good, bad, and ugly. It is forced upon us. You can't go back, so be open and receptive to starting anew with enlightenment and an awareness of the divine teachers that will keep coming into your life. Have faith in destiny's design.

Sending you strength, love, and trust.

Love,
Mom

Enlightenment

"Whatever you do will be insignificant, but it is very important that you do it." –Gandhi

Hearing the initial news from my daughter of her anal cancer diagnosis, I was forced to refocus. Everything else in my life became unequivocally insignificant. So my new revolved life began.

I found strength in the help of family and friends. I was there for my daughter in any and every way I could be such as comforting gifts, emails, phone calls, medical knowledge, and words of nurturing endearments. Focusing on my own physical and mental strengths helped me cope. Yoga, meditating, journaling, walking, exercising, healthy eating, relaxing music, aromatherapy, and spiritual readings were essential self-care practices. To help her, I had to put myself first. I had to stay well, physically and mentally, in order to be strong for her.

By practicing self-care, self-compassion, and accepting the help from family and friends, I felt an intense, loving nature develop inside of me. My soul and a higher power have been activated. Our number one relationship should be with the creative spiritual energy of God (our source, our purpose, our truth). I trust inspiration is always there for me when needed.

I am happy to say Angela's results came back November 28, 2017, and she is now cancer-free. She has returned to work. Angela and I have both been through a lot. We will never be the same. I feel a sense of peace and hope within me. Now and forever enlightened consciousness will always be our guide.

****

REFERENCES:

Brown, Brene (2010). The Power of Vulnerability, TEDx (video). https://www.ted.com/talks/brene_brown_on_vulnerability/up-next

Brown, Brene (2012). *Daring Greatly: How the Courage to Be Vulnerable Transforms the Way We Live, Love, Parent, and Lead.* USA: Penguin Publishing Group.

Tolle, Eckhart (2006). *A New Earth: Awakening to Your Life's Purpose.* USA: Penguin Book.

Weil, Andrew (1995). *Spontaneous Healing: How to Discover and Enhance Your Body's Natural Ability to Maintain and Heal Itself.* New York: Knopf.

Chapter 21

"Anal_Cancer Support" Facebook Group

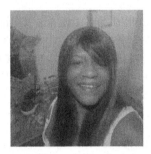

An Interview with Maria L. Barr: Founder of the
Anal_Cancer Support group on Facebook

Angela G. Gentile: *Can you share a little bit about yourself and your anal cancer experience?*

Maria L. Barr: In January 2007, I was having some intermittent pain and light bleeding in my anal region. Since I had diabetes, I was seeing my doctor every three months for A1C tests. I mentioned the bleeding and thought it might be hemorrhoids. I wasn't too concerned. As months went by, however, the pain and bleeding got worse, and I began having trouble doing number two. I was getting scared and becoming more and more alarmed.

In June of 2007, I made an appointment with my doctor to find out what was happening. She took one look and said, "That's not a hemorrhoid." She sent me immediately to a surgeon who had an office in the building. He took one look and scheduled me for a biopsy.

I will never forget the day the results came back. I sat opposite him in his office at his desk, and he told me it was "Squamous Cell Carcinoma—Anal Cancer."

My response was "How do we get rid of it?" All I wanted at that moment was for it to be GONE. We discussed my options: remove it surgically and end up with a colostomy bag or treat with both chemotherapy and radiation. I was 38 years old, and the thought of a colostomy bag was out of the question. So, I opted for chemo and radiation.

In July of 2007, I started treatments which included 28 days straight of radiation and two weeks of chemotherapy. My iron was low, so first I had to get my iron levels up. I was hospitalized for my chemo. It took four days to get all of the chemo in me, and I was transported by ambulance to my radiation appointments. In October of 2007, I was declared cancer-free.

In March of 2008, I had a recurrence. I went to the Sylvester Cancer Center in Miami for a second opinion. The doctor there agreed with the cancer board and my team for more aggressive chemotherapy and radiation. They felt I could handle it. This time I had 14 days of radiation twice a day and four rounds of chemotherapy every three weeks. I had them implant a port because my veins suffered greatly the first time.

My oncologist wanted to start right away, but I had tickets to go on a cruise to Mexico in May, and I didn't want to be on a cruise ship between treatments. I was feeling well at the time and didn't believe that starting treatment right away would make that big of a difference. I had a great time on the cruise.

In June 2008, I started treatments again. It was much worse than the first time around. I continued working as much as I could. I would go to radiation in the morning before work, then leave work early to go to radiation again before going home for the day. Each round of chemo was a hospital stay with me begging to go home as soon as it was done. I had to stay if I was too dehydrated. My boss was very understanding and even paid for me to have Healing Touch therapy while I was going through treatments. I had so much

216

trouble with food that I borrowed a juicer from a friend and made fresh vegetable and fruit juices when I couldn't eat.

Where are you at now in your cancer experience?

I am living with the horrible side effects of treatment. I do not have healthcare insurance at the moment and haven't been able to visit a doctor. I eat healthily and take good care of myself.

Describe the time when you decided to start a group for those affected by anal cancer. Also, tell us how it grew.

Once I was given my diagnosis, I went on the Internet looking for anything I could find about anal cancer. There was so much information about all kinds of cancer, but all I could find on anal cancer were medical research papers and articles in medical journals. There was some information on the American Cancer Society website and the National Cancer Institute, but not much. I found a website called CarePages (which is now shut down). It was like a Facebook for sick people. It made it easy to let friends and family know how I was doing. That's where I met Joana Dougherty McGee. She gave me such valuable advice on dealing with side effects of treatment. I also found a forum for rare cancers but found it difficult to navigate. In February 2009, I decided to create the ANAL CANCER Facebook group (now called Anal_Cancer Support) to provide a place for others like me who wanted to share stories and advice. I never had to promote the group. It has grown on its own.

Did you encounter any problems or issues with the group?

Anal_Cancer Support started out as an open group, and there were a lot of members. Some people were posting things that were inappropriate, and some posted advertisements. I had to clean it up by removing some members and blocking others. I also had to change it to a closed group (posts visible only to members) and added a questionnaire for those seeking membership.

What have the members said about being in the group?

I have had minimal complaints about other members since making the group closed. A few members have stated they were happy they found the group.

What motivates you to continue to administer the group?

I love seeing people supporting each other. I feel the group is needed, and as long as even just one person finds comfort there, I will keep it up. It's nice to communicate with people who know what you are going through. I couldn't find much of that years ago.

Who would most benefit from joining the group?

Anyone touched by anal cancer in need of support and camaraderie.

Is there a screening process? Who is eligible to join?

Three questions need to be answered before I accept a member request. I only did that to weed out the trolls (people just looking to create trouble). People diagnosed with cancer, family members, and caregivers are all welcome.

Describe who makes up the membership.

Currently, we have a diverse group of over 170 members, and our group is growing (unfortunately). We have members from the US, UK, Canada, Mexico, and other parts of the world. Two-thirds of our membership is female, and one-third is male. We do not screen for sexual orientation, and we do have some openly homosexual members.

What are your plans for the group?

We have changed the name from ANAL CANCER to Anal_Cancer Support, and I have added moderators. We are the only professionally moderated anal cancer group on Facebook that I am aware of. I would like to do more with the group and am open to suggestions.

> Support and strength can be gained by participating in a professionally moderated or led support group. (*cancer.gov*)

How can people find the group?

Search Facebook groups for "Anal_Cancer Support" or go to *facebook.com/groups/analcancersupport/*.

Any other supports out there you could recommend to people with anal cancer?

I joined Gilda's Club in South Florida. It's an awesome support group affiliated with the Cancer Support Community.

Anything else you want to share?

I believe information and education are essential to prevent deaths from anal cancer. No one should die from this disease.

Thank you, Maria! You are doing great work. Keep it up!

Chapter 22

Advocating for Change

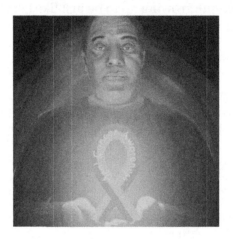

Calvin Nokes

I never thought depression and anxiety would affect me, but here I am. I have been suffering for years. I battled depression and struggled with being gay since I was a teenager. The fact that I live in a world with Donald Trump as the U.S. President causes me added stressors and mood problems. This man is really bad for my immune system.

I have had some serious health scares. I was diagnosed HIV positive in 1988. HIV (human immunodeficiency virus) causes acquired immune deficiency syndrome, also known as AIDS. I was also diagnosed with not only one, but two cancers in 2009, including anal cancer.

I will share my experiences with three serious medical diagnoses, my treatment for them, and my resultant emotional upheaval including depression and anxiety. I will also describe my current advocacy and volunteer work, and how I overcame anal cancer. Ultimately, I want to help increase awareness of anal cancer and help people survive it.

The HIV Diagnosis

Growing up in a Christian family, I always felt unloved and alienated. As a young boy, there was a woman who was transsexual who babysat me. I didn't know what transsexual was, but I heard people joke about me growing up to be just like her. I was confused. I loved this woman. I struggled with my sexual orientation for many years. I was told by a therapist I had experienced a lot of spiritual abuse.

I didn't speak much with God. I felt he too was disappointed in me, so I sought out comfort in substance abuse. I got addicted to drugs and alcohol, and I began acting out sexually. This was the beginning of a self-destructive pattern. I was looking for love. I was looking in the wrong places, by drinking and having unprotected sex with anonymous men.

Hearing the news that I was HIV positive hurt pretty bad. There were not many nice things being said about gays at that time. It was not much of a surprise given how I was acting out at the time. I remember feeling at a loss and not knowing what to do. So, I called my mom, and all she said was "Oh well." I wasn't sure how to take that, but in retrospect, what could she have said?

However, I was blessed to be in the right place, and I was connected with some amazing people. I started my medicines, and they seemed to work well. Unfortunately, they started to upset my stomach. I was switched to another regimen, but either my compliance slipped or the blood work was not good. The drugs were changed about four times.

Fast-forward to 30 years later. I am on the last available regimen that is currently recommended. I am not giving up, and I consistently get my blood counts checked. Thus far, the numbers are good. There are days I want to forget my medicines after taking them for decades. I'm usually pretty good at taking them but do worry about the long-term consequences of continual use.

Getting the So-Called Hemorrhoid Checked Out

Let's go back to 2009. June 25th of that year is a day I promise never to forget. Everyone was talking about the loss of Michael Jackson, the "King of Pop," and not much was being said about the death of Farrah Fawcett (American actress and pin-up model) who died of anal cancer the same day. I was crushed. It also caused me anxiety.

While all this was happening, I was seeing my doctor for what I was hoping was just a hemorrhoid. I had them when I was younger, but this time the so-called hemorrhoid was getting bigger, and I also noticed blood. I knew it was time to get it checked out.

I had a biopsy about the time of my 50th birthday that year. My best friend went with me to lend support. The surgeon asked me if I knew what procedure I was in for during my surgery preparation. My friend and I both agreed we hoped they knew what they were supposed to do. The doctor said he was just confirming with me. The procedure was quick, and I was on my way home in about two hours.

Devastating News

After 21 years of surviving HIV, I got the biggest scare of my life. I was so excited to turn 50 because I never thought I would make it. That excitement didn't last long because a week later I was diagnosed with anal cancer.

I remember the day I was told I had anal cancer. The weather was beautiful. I was a little tense, not knowing what I would hear. When the doctor came in, he just said, "Mr. Nokes, you have cancer." It felt as though the air got sucked out of the room. After that, I heard nothing more.

I remember leaving the office and talking to myself. "Did the doctor just say I had cancer?" I was in disbelief, and I remembered crying in his office when he said something about surgery and a possible colostomy bag (a receptacle which collects feces that comes out of an opening in the abdominal wall). It was a very long walk back to the subway station, and the ride was even more insane. I burst into tears. I kept trying to convince myself this wasn't real.

Finding information specific to anal cancer was difficult. I could not find an active support group, but I do, fortunately, have the support of friends. This lack of information left me a little irate and made me determined to improve this situation for other people.

I was devastated, and at the same time, I was grieving the loss of Farrah. I just adored her, and I had no idea how to deal with her loss and having the same cancer that took her life. I was convinced I, too, was going to die.

I had additional imaging. If all that wasn't bad enough, a week later I was told I also had another cancer called Hodgkin lymphoma. Anxiety kicked into overdrive. I was thinking to myself, "This is not good. After all, I'm HIV positive." I hadn't digested the fact I had anal cancer, and all I could think of was this was my fault. I couldn't shake the fact I lost a favorite celebrity to the same cancer.

My head was working overtime, mainly thinking I was going to die. I cried a lot. I played the blame game. I felt everything was my fault. I screamed at my partner. Nothing was right. I went "off the wall." I ended up with stomach issues, and I felt wound up all the time. I couldn't shake it. I was in so much pain psychologically and emotionally. I became run-down, and my immune system was susceptible to all kinds of germs.

Cancer Treatments Started

Farrah's death hit me hard. I remember hearing she wanted to keep her cancer diagnosis private, but for a celebrity, privacy wasn't in the cards for her. The cancer that took her was considered rare, and very little was known about it. She even tried some alternative medicine. I started my treatments as early as possible and was fortunate Medicare (a federal health insurance plan in the U.S.A.) assured my access and continuity of care.

My radiation treatments were an adventure in and of themselves. There was an hour going to and from the hospital, and all the time I spent waiting. I had an old friend taking me to most of my appointments, and ironically, I was diagnosed on his birthday, July 27th. His pick-up truck had heated seats, and that was a blessing sometimes given how my posterior was aching.

I can recall a lot of pain starting on the third or fourth radiation treatment. I had to wear Depends® (disposable adult incontinence briefs). I learned about sitz baths. At first, I disliked them because it was so raw back there—but once I got used to them, they were heavenly. I dreaded being too far from a toilet as accidents did happen.

My thoughts were in overdrive. I tried to laugh it off, but I felt small. I felt the ordeal would never be over. Then the tears came, and it felt like I could fill buckets.

I also remember lots of walking and my partner trying to encourage me that the exercise was good for me. It turns out he was right. I knew I had to watch what I ate, and things like fried chicken were not recommended. Unfortunately, my one friend acting as my caregiver liked chili. My system and butt weren't too appreciative of that. I can't complain too much as he was the one who ensured I attended my chemotherapy treatment, which occurred on weekends.

My chemotherapy was provided over several weekends about a month after radiation treatment began. This was done in the hospital after being admitted and given IV drips of chemotherapy agents. This was due in part as a regimen to treat the anal cancer and the Hodgkin lymphoma. It worked but made me miserable the whole time and days afterwards. Bedpans and I became very familiar on those weekends.

I was fortunate to have my partner support me the whole time I was in and out of the hospital for tests and treatment. He always made sure I made it to my appointments. When he wasn't available (because he works full-time), he arranged a ride for me. He hosted me at his house, so I did not have to worry about meals, laundry, and running for prescriptions. He tried to entertain me with gallows humor (grim or ironic humor in a desperate situation) and hogging the TV remote. I was able to rest when the pain let me.

The Emotional and Physical Lows

I experienced so many feelings. The strongest one was depression. I felt like I was dying. I thought to myself, "After all, I am HIV positive, so how much luck can I count on? I am not a cat with nine lives." Also, I was sort of a "bad" patient. I was still smoking cigarettes, and my attitude was "I have two cancers already, so screw it." I sort of regret that now, but the good news is I quit in 2011, as hard as that was to stop.

I was lucky I was able to receive enough painkillers to help cope with the side effects of the treatment. I was also prescribed antianxiety medicine. These took the edge off but just that. I hate to contemplate what it would be like nine years later with all the new concerns and restrictions on opioids.

I was lucky to be caught at stage 1 with both cancers. All my worrying was wasted energy because I survived both cancers, and I've lived 30 years with HIV.

Advocating Since 2010

I have been advocating for anal cancer since early 2010. I volunteer for the American Cancer Society as well as the American Cancer Society Cancer Action Network (ACS CAN). I have two Facebook groups I monitor, and I help by sharing my story with others. We truly need more awareness because when I was diagnosed there was scant information available. I help fundraise and attend events including ACS CAN Lobby Day. The Lights of Hope display every year is a high point of the event. We visit with members of Congress to advocate for funding for treatment, and to lobby for new legislation responsive to people diagnosed with cancer and for survivors' needs.

When I was diagnosed, it was difficult to find anything about anal cancer. As I mentioned previously, the lack of information was very upsetting. I remember coming back from my diagnosis appointment and looking up anal cancer. I was amazed and so outraged I couldn't find much on the subject. Even today some cancer sites do not include anal cancer.

This is not acceptable, especially if we are working on eliminating the associated stigma. It seems there are a lot of people who don't like to talk about anything related to our anus. Maybe they think it's dirty? I never understood that because if something doesn't seem right, I'm getting it checked out. I don't care what body part it is. Folks need to know that this cancer exists, and it is serious. Anal cancer is nothing to be ashamed of or embarrassed about.

To help end the stigma, I continue working with ACS CAN and tell my story whenever there is someone who will listen. If I find anal cancer missing from a website or other cancer resource, I contact the source and encourage them to add the information. I also help advocate and support the need for teaching young people and their parents the importance of the HPV vaccine and safer sex practices. Prevention is also an essential part of ending the stigma.

Palliative Care is Not Just for the Terminally Ill

Palliative care is one of the things I learned about through my lobbying work with ACS CAN. Palliative care is not just about caring for those with cancer who are terminal but about providing care for the whole person. It is care focused on providing relief from the symptoms and stress of a serious illness. The goal is to improve the quality of life for both the patient and the family.

Palliative care was one of the things I was sorely lacking. The doctors were taking care of my body but did little to ease my mind or my concerns. They recommended support groups, but none of them had a standing schedule when I was undergoing treatment.

It is a privilege to be associated with ACS CAN and to continue advocating. I visit and try to speak with my members of Congress by sharing my story. I could have benefited from appropriate palliative care mentally and spiritually as I endured chemotherapy and radiation treatments.

I'm thrilled that I helped ACS CAN get a bill passed for palliative care. It's called the H.R. 1676–Palliative Care and Hospice

Education and Training Act. I am also thrilled to have been featured in an advertisement for the American Cancer Society. This ad was in the paper while I was attending Lobby Day in Washington D.C. I have supported Relay for Life fundraising events, especially the Survivor Walks. As a survivor, I want to make it easier for others to cope with the stress and trauma cancer brings.

Advocating is my Mission

When I was diagnosed, I had no problem saying I had anal cancer. Why should I? It was not like I had a choice of what cancer I got. Even though I was diagnosed with two cancers, I focus more on the anal cancer because it was practically unknown except for the fact that a celebrity had just lost her life from it.

Every day I will be advocating anal cancer awareness; that is my mission. Most people I speak to have never heard of anal cancer. I barely had until I was diagnosed. However, I vividly remember Farrah and the news back then. I also ensure people are aware of World Anal Cancer Awareness Day—March 21st. I will continue to advocate for anal cancer awareness and patient support.

Cancer research is important to me for a personal reason, primarily because it provided the knowledge that resulted in my effective treatment. I was shocked and scared when I was diagnosed, but I trusted the medical personnel who treated me to do the right thing. It worked, and I am currently cancer-free. I want to help ensure others have a similar positive outcome.

I know some people still feel uncomfortable talking about anal cancer. I am heavily involved in forums on Facebook. I even nicknamed myself the "Assbassador" for Anal Cancer Awareness. But, seriously, I am determined to advocate for cancer awareness and treatment. I especially want to raise awareness about anal cancer. Not a week goes by that I don't address the concern of anal cancer.

Anal Cancer Ribbon

One thing I am proud of is helping to get a unique ribbon for anal cancer warriors and survivors (much like breast cancer has the pink ribbon). There was a petition, and it took off. The HPV and Anal Cancer Foundation partnered with the Farrah Fawcett Foundation on this project. The colors chosen for the anal cancer ribbon were purple and green. The ribbon can be found on The HPV and Anal Cancer Foundation website and is available for downloading and using wherever needed to help spread awareness.

Staying Positive

I have so much to be thankful for. I have to work at having a positive mindset continually. I'm trying to do just this—stay positive, count my blessings, and rise up every morning to say "Thank you God" for all I have. Sometimes I have to say to myself, "Get with the program!" I'm fortunate, and I'm often told by people I share my story with that I should run to church, fall on my knees, and humbly thank Him.

My anxiety and depression are managed well by seeing a psychotherapist on a regular basis, and I also take Prozac, an antidepressant medication. My partner, who loves me through the good and bad, helps keep me in check. I also love my cat, my gospel music, and going on long walks.

For those diagnosed with anal cancer, I want you to know there is hope for survival and recovery. You may need to accept a new normal temporarily. It's not easy, but know feeling bad is going to happen. Keep working through it and try to be sure to have a support network to help you cope. When you come out on the other side, focus on the future. Look forward to how you can do better and maybe like me you can give back to others as part of your gratitude.

****

RESOURCES:

American Cancer Society Cancer Action Network
(*acscan.org*)

Anal Cancer It's a Pain in the Butt Literally (Facebook page)
(*facebook.com/AnalCancerRibbonPage/*)

The Farrah Fawcett Foundation
(*thefarrahfawcettfoundation.org*)

The HPV and Anal Cancer Foundation
(*analcancerfoundation.org*)

Chapter 23

Life Lessons:
What CANCER Taught Me

Laura Zick-Mauzy

LIFE ...

Available for a limited time only. Limited to one (1) per person. Non-transferrable—no warranty. Subject to change without notice. Terms and conditions do apply. There is no owner's manual. Life is fragile. Handle with care. Expiration date indeterminate.

Much to my surprise, cancer <u>taught</u> me things.

I didn't expect that.

But, I've seen my life change. I've seen my priorities and my attitude change. That has filled me with awe. I'm in my 50s, and I never imagined at this point in my life I'd have my world turned upside down and have that turn out to be a good thing. ☺

Cancer has taught me . . .

- **To pursue deep <u>emotional connections</u> with people.**

I find myself being interested on a different level. I want to

CONNECT with people . . . to be real . . . to be available . . .

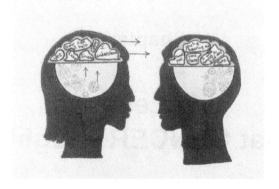

*A drawing of how I perceive myself being
more available.*

- **To _experience_ dreams, not just dream them.**

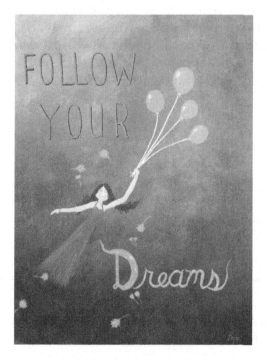

*I painted this to remind myself (and others)
to follow (y)our dreams.*

Whenever possible, I am taking chances. I've always dreamed of traveling after I retire. I really wanted to see the Grand Canyon, for example. But, I realized, I do not need to wait until I retire. None of us know how long we're on this earth, so why wait for my dreams to happen . . . Why not MAKE them happen? So, that's what I'm doing. I went to the Grand Canyon this year, and I look forward to future adventures.

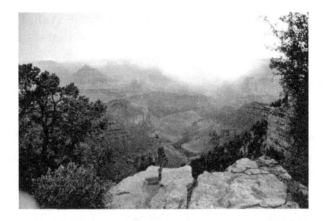

Grand Canyon, 2015

- **To <u>reach out</u> to other patients.**

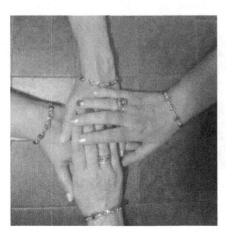

I work in the medical field. I care about people. After having cancer, there's a deeper level of caring. It's hard to explain, it's just . . . deeper. I've been "meeting" people through my blog, and I've learned there's camaraderie amongst survivors. I am blessed to be meeting people who have experienced the same struggles, treatments, side effects, and emotions. I've learned to reach out . . .

- **To take opportunities, <u>just because</u>.**

There have been things in my life that I've had the opportunity to do but chose not to because they didn't seem that important, were too intimidating, or they just weren't "me." I'm taking those opportunities now. Here's an example: my employer has an annual gala, and it's a fundraiser . . . one of those events for the uppity-ups to get together and rub elbows. Everyone is invited to get dressed up, and "everyone who is someone" will be there. Well, I went this year. Yep, me—who is so far from an "uppity-up" that it's not funny. Why?

Why not? I had the opportunity. And I took it, just because . . .

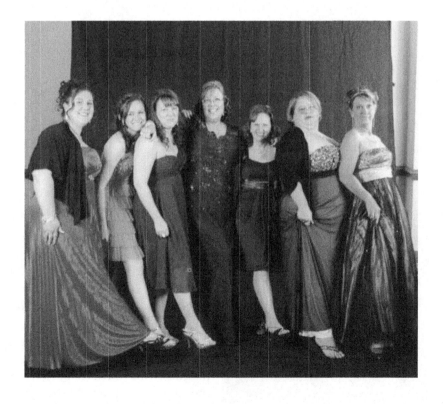

That's me in the center. Out of scrubs and into a gown.

- **To prioritize <u>differently</u>.**

I can prioritize, no problems there. I just do it differently now. Things I fretted over (before cancer) aren't worth my worry now. If everything doesn't get ironed on Tuesday, so what? If I failed to pull weeds, who cares? If I'm not able to cook tonight, it's not a big deal. My husband had been trying to convince me these things are trivial, that I shouldn't stress about them. I just didn't seem to be able to adopt that attitude. Cancer changed that. It's taught me to enjoy each day. I still prioritize, just differently. If something doesn't get done, it's okay; tomorrow is another day and EACH day should have joy . . .

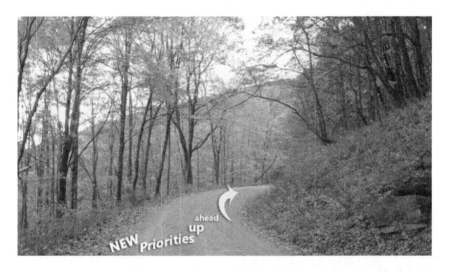

Priorities have changed.

- **To become more <u>purpose</u>-driven.**

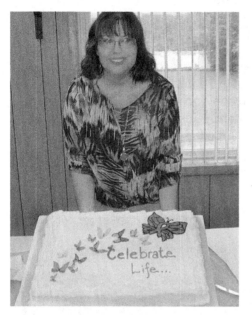

I'm living life with purpose now. Every day is a gift, and I appreciate that gift. I set more short-term goals now. They're not large, unattainable goals, but rather they're little things that mean something (to me or to someone else). It is life . . . Celebrate it!

- **To express <u>love</u> more openly.**

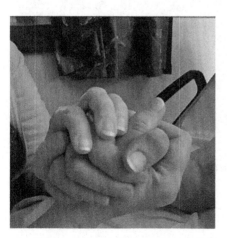

I say "I love you" more frequently. I tell my family. I tell my friends. I want to live without regret. I want to apologize when needed and show love as often as possible. Kindness truly does matter . . . Show it . . . Mean it.

Holding someone's hand can mean holding their heart.

- **To <u>relax</u>.**

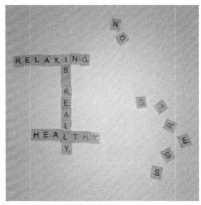

I've been through a lot of polar opposites in my life. I've been extremely thin and extremely overweight. I've had a lot of money and hardly enough to live on. I've been loved and resented. I've been tremendously respected and had times of being looked down upon. My health is more important than any of those things, and I needed to exhale and not be so uptight. Cancer has taught me that my identity is not in any of the above. I can relax and just be me. I can relax and just be . . .

- **To go beyond my <u>comfort zone</u>.**

Writing was WAY beyond my comfort zone. I'm putting some very personal things out there in public that I thought I would NEVER share, even with family members, ever . . . But, I've grown and learned, and that's an awesome thing. I'm moving outside the box; moving past the stigma was somewhat painful, but moving outside my comfort zone in other areas of my life has been so rewarding. I am LIVING life. I have begun painting, drove bumper cars with my granddaughter (yes, that was actually a big deal), went to Disney World and New York City, opened a photography studio, and many MANY other things I thought I would never do. . . . things I thought I COULD NEVER DO.

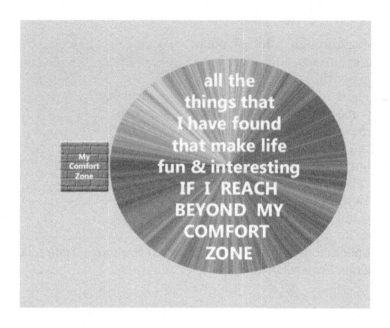

So, I have had some meaningful life lessons come out of my cancer journey—and those I would not trade for anything.

****

Adapted from "Life Lessons. What CANCER Taught Me," Anal About Cancer (blog), by Laura Zick-Mauzy, April 5, 2014. (analaboutcancer.com)

Chapter 24

"Anal Cancer Help" Website

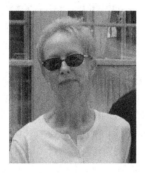

Marshall Carter-Tripp

AnalCancerHelp.info

Some eight years ago I discovered a small anal polyp, and a biopsy characterized it as "squamous cell anal carcinoma." More discoveries followed, such as the widespread reluctance to use the word "anal," and the belief that anyone so diagnosed must have engaged in "kinky sex." The only person I knew who shared this cancer was told by her radiologist, in the presence of her adult son, "anal cancer is the result of anal sex." She was so ashamed that she refused to tell anyone she was undergoing cancer treatment to prevent anyone from asking what kind of cancer she had!

Internet searches turned up few if any resources for anal cancer patients and no focused websites at all. So I set to work to create one, "Anal Cancer Help" (*analcancerhelp.info*), pulling together as many reliable medical sites as possible (e.g., no links to sites promising cures or prevention by eating rose petals). I have a Ph.D., and I am familiar with research procedures and evaluations. The website is seasoned with humor and nutrition advice, and I have made the site as comprehensive and useful as possible. The opening pages describe anal cancer and the shift in treating it—from immediate anal surgery that generally resulted in an ostomy bag—to a one-two punch of radiation and chemotherapy, in a short but brutal six-week period.

Ladies: Dab! —Don't Wipe!

The key to understanding anal cancer is the relatively new knowledge of the human papillomavirus, or HPV. We now know nearly everyone is infected with this virus, and certain strains of it are responsible for most cervical and anal cancers, along with vulvar and penile cancers. HPV moves effortlessly between the anal and genital areas, and despite reporting focused on men having sex with men, anal sex is not the only way to contract an HPV infection. For example, there are indications that improperly cleaned surgical tools may transfer it. For women, "wiping from front to back" can spread the virus. So ladies—dab, don't wipe!

It is crucial for those who receive an anal cancer diagnosis to avoid giving in to a sense of shame and perpetuating the stigma, which may well prevent others from seeking help if they suspect something is wrong "down there." AND it is also important that doctors do not dismiss anal polyps as "just hemorrhoids," and they do not avoid touching their patients (in the digital rectal exam). Anal cancer is rare compared to most other cancers in the US, and even some oncologists are not familiar with it—so you may have to be your own research expert and advocate!

Humor can help relieve the stress of diagnosis and treatment, and often it can be the best medicine. Once I started to compile "rear end" cartoons, I was surprised to discover how much was out there. For example, I found a greeting card (at the grocery store!) that showed three planets lined up and the middle one says to the front one "I can see Uranus!" Open up the card, and it states, "You're never too old for butt jokes! Happy birthday!" If you take a look at the "funny stuff" page on the website, you will see many more.

I have received dozens of emails via my website asking for help of various kinds or just generally commenting, some from outside the US such as Canada, Australia, and the UK. Clearly, there is still a lack of information and help out there. I will keep it online and update it with new material as long as I can.

Chapter 25

Conclusion

Angela G. Gentile

*The word anthology comes from the Greek anthologia which
means a "collection of flowers."*

There are many voices to be heard. Some are loud, some are
quiet. Some speak from a place of shame, others speak from
a loving place deep within their hearts. Educating voices
strive to teach. Sharing voices endeavor to heal. The advocates are
persistent. The common threads that run through these voices are
strength, hope, and courage.

Whether we are affected by anal cancer personally, or as a friend or
family member, we all have an important message to share. Putting
this all into a book format has made it permanent. *Cancer Up the
Wazoo* will be available forever. It is a legacy that we leave behind.
Something we pass along to those who come after us. We aspire to
plant seeds of hope for the future.

Writing for and editing this book has been a therapeutic process for
me. Many of the contributing writers are first-time published
authors. It was a pleasure and joy for me to coach, encourage,
support and inspire these amazing people. I've grown leaps and
bounds in terms of my own personal growth. These courageous,
inspiring, and loving men and women have moved and energized
me. I feel better and stronger as a result of them sharing their
stories and experiences. My heart is full.

All the contributors and I thank you for reading. Thank you for helping us in our quest to end the stigma of having anal cancer. We are happy to share our stories, provide information and offer hope. We ask that when you are finished with this collection, please pass it along to someone else who you think may need it. Whether it's to learn something new, offer some enlightenment, or provide resources to help them cope with their own cancer experience. It takes a village to help one cope with cancer. Thank you for being part of our village.

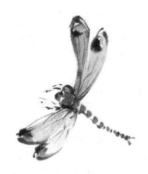

Chapter 26

Epilogue

Angela G. Gentile

Joy Anderson: "It has been over three years since the surgery to remove the cancer, over two since the last chemo. There have been other issues, but the cancer seems to be gone. For the most part, my life is back on track. I live on five acres that I inherited from my parents, that I am fixing up. One of the projects is what I am calling my "Witch Shack." It will be a spot to work on my hobbies, painting, sewing, herbs, etc. I have also continued my other passion, as festival director of a group I belong to called Earth Spirit People (earthspiritpeople.org). We have at least two major gatherings a year where we have speakers, workshops, music, drumming, sweat lodge and rituals. I have been involved in this for over ten years and was still doing it during my treatments. I am changing some of the things that I was doing. I have let my livestock, except for chickens, go. I am now officially retired and plan to work more on my art and spiritual projects. I have always had an appreciation for life, but going through all this has made it more so. I have learned to slow down a bit and appreciate what I have and the beauty around me."

Maria L. Barr currently doesn't have medical insurance and hasn't been to a doctor in years. She eats a healthy diet and takes good care of herself. She recently celebrated her 10th anniversary of completing treatments.

Sharon Basic is currently three years from treatment and doing very well. So far no evidence of cancer. She has to deal with some side effects from treatment, but they are manageable. She is very thankful to have had terrific care from her oncologists, surgeon, family doctor, CAREpath nurse, family and friends.

Peggy Belton remains NED (no evidence of disease) and lives what appears to be a normal life on the outside. Like most, she struggles with the late effects of radiation and the voice of fear in the back of her mind. Her goldendoodle puppy helps keep her focus on the joy of today.

Michael DeHart: "I did receive standard Nigro protocol—5FU + mitomycin + radiation therapy (chemoradiation). I had two additional radiation treatments at the end so I would qualify for a clinical trial testing the effectiveness of Nivolumab on preventing anal cancer recurrence. Nivolumab is an immunotherapy drug—an exciting class of new treatments that are quickly becoming a standard of care in cancer treatment. Nivolumab works as a checkpoint inhibitor, which blocks a chemical signal that usually tells t-cells not to attack your cancer. I'm praying that I'm in the arm of the study that gets the drug.

I had concerns about peripheral neuropathy being more difficult after receiving mitomycin, and that has become more of a problem. Unfortunately, I've had to increase my dosage of gabapentin (Neurontin) to combat my now increased peripheral neuropathy.

It's now been ten weeks since I finished treatment, and I am working full-time again. This is only possible because I work from home for myself, but I do put in 8-10 hour days. I'm just now starting to think about the gym again. While what I went through was incredibly difficult and frightening, I'm incredibly grateful to have a third chance at life (as this was my second time with cancer). Now I focus on doing everything I can to prevent recurrence, even though my oncologist told me he feels my chances of recurrence are very low. In addition to my Nivolumab clinical trial, I use a high-quality liposomal curcumin product (turmeric extract), which has

246

shown to have potent anticancer properties in multiple studies with very little toxicity at doses required to fight cancer.

Joana Dougherty McGee is now over 12 years out of treatment and continues to be free of cancer. Her treatment resulted in permanent, everyday complications from pelvic radiation disease, something that was an expected eventuality, due to pre-existing conditions that jeopardized treatment toleration. She was unable to return to work on a regular basis but continues to independently educate and counsel, both online and, with limited hours, in the community.

At present, along with the founding colleague (Maria L. Barr) and the author of this book, Angela. G. Gentile, she co-administers a Facebook support group for patients (and caregivers of patients) dealing with anal cancer.

Through Joana's extensive experience working with children who have cancer, she feels that she was given an incomparable gift of perspective, which made her own cancer(s) experience considerably more tolerable to submit to and endure, both physically and emotionally. "Overwhelmingly, they come to grasp the precious nature of life and love intuitively," she says, "and whenever they are healthy enough to celebrate it, they do. They are grateful, and they're wise—really; they possess such grace and dignity."

She and her husband are in the process of moving permanently to Cantabria, Spain. Her pipe dream is to write the many books she has inside her head and heart. Among countless other things, she is passionate about music/playing/singing; animals; the environment; humor; social justice; crafting, and, alas, grammar (the latter making her husband's eyes glaze over!)!

Jodi Canaday Green is a public school administrator and has continued to be cancer free since January of 2014. She continues to see her oncology surgeon, medical oncologist, and radiation oncologist. Even though she will continue to experience some very unpleasant side effect from treatment, she considers herself blessed. She spends her days appreciating and loving her family and works hard to educate others on the signs and symptoms of anal cancer.

Virginia Lloyd-Davies: "When I was going through anal cancer chemo-radiation in 2016, I didn't think I would survive it. What kept me going was my painting. Some images were dark and desperate; others showed my determination to let the light in. On the days when I couldn't walk the 50 steps to my studio, at least I could paint in my imagination.

Nearly two years later, I find that my painting is growing in depth and boldness as I listen to my inner voice rather than the world's expectations. I followed the rules of Chinese brush painting for decades; now my brush follows my heart."

Calvin Nokes: "Since writing my chapter earlier this year, I have passed several milestones. I managed to abstain from drugs and alcohol for the last month and hope to continue that trend. I celebrated my 59th birthday with dinner out sans alcohol. Yesterday marked 24.5 years with my partner who has stood by my side (mostly) during my arduous journey. And just as significantly, I passed my ninth cancerversary, and I am grateful to have done so."

Sheila Roy: "Wow so much time has passed by, and I am finally able to breathe a sigh and realize that the nightmare is over and Angela is doing really well. It's a scary feeling. So hopeful, yet feeling the sting and worry from before. I look at Angela and am joyful to see the vibrant, ambitious and kind person we all know, is back. It's like getting the best news; on the one hand worried, anxious . . . but now so happy and so relieved. It changed my life and how I view things now. Every day is a gift, and every gift needs to be enjoyed to the fullest, and we need to give thanks for all our blessings. Life is good."

Alan S. Wolkenstein: "While it has been over twenty years since the diagnosis of cancer, I can say that 'the view from my window' has changed dramatically. I had been lost, a traveler who was thrown by the diagnosis to the ends of the earth. The trip back has been difficult, challenging, and wondrous.

I sensed immediately the losses that occurred to me physically, spiritually, and emotionally. After a time, I realized that life needed to be more than grieving and lamenting these losses that occurred with little to no respite in-between. If I was to live, really live, I needed to seek and then find purpose and meaning to my life—and I found it. With help from my family and friends, therapy, spirituality and just plain luck, I found my way back. And life is yet so expansive and encompassing, as it should be. I am blessed. The view is spectacular."

Laura Zick-Mauzy: "Today I had (what should've been) my last oncology appointment. I'll still have yearly colonoscopies until there aren't any tubular adenomas found. I'm a superhero at making those. I also learned things after five years that STUNNED ME. Although I was "told" I was stage 1, the cancer was aggressive, and a tiny lymph node lit up on the PET scan. I knew that part. It was needle biopsied and was negative. But, because the node was such a small one, my oncologist never considered it confirmed OR RULED OUT. So, . . . I was treated as if my cancer was a stage 3a. The five-year survival rate for 3a is 48%. If the polyp hadn't been found in the routine colonoscopy, it would likely have metastasized. I would probably be dead now. But she found it, so it didn't. And I am an anal cancer warrior—now penning my own personal journey through this disease that attempted to take me down."

And for me, **Angela G. Gentile**, I am truly grateful and honored to have been the catalyst for *Cancer Up the Wazoo*. One-year post-treatment, I am thriving and enjoying life—living life to the fullest, for I do not know how much time I have left in this wonderful life. I am honored to have been able to "listen to," edit and share these stories and very happy to call all of the contributors friends. We share an indelible bond, and for that, I am genuinely thankful. My life is enriched due to this cancer experience.

Appendix A

Self-Affirmations

Angela G. Gentile
with Professor Alan S. Wolkenstein (a.k.a. Prof)

"I lovingly forgive and release all of the past. I choose to fill
my world with joy. I love and approve of myself."
–Louise Hay healing affirmation for cancer

Our fears and anxieties can be a direct result of our negative
thinking. Positive thinking can help allay our fears and worries. We
should acknowledge our fears and concerns are important;
however, remaining stuck in that place is not good for our mental
and physical health. It can cause us stress, and this can negatively
impact our overall well-being.

Self-affirmations are positive statements that are self-empowering.
Repeating them to yourself either silently in your mind, or out loud,
can help shift your mind and body into a state of well-being. Prof
states, "Saying them out loud gives your mind and spirit permission
to hear and reverberate with the energy released."

Find a quiet place and still your body and mind. Some say doing the
exercise in front of a mirror has an even more powerful effect. Take
a few deep breaths first. Even though you may not fully believe the
statements, saying them as if you do will help your subconscious
thoughts move toward a state of well-being. We know you don't
have to fully believe in the statement to gain benefit. These
affirmations can be done any time of day or night and can be said
any number of times during the day.

To start, we suggest selecting (or writing your own) five statements,
then expand as you are ready. Recite these statements at least twice
daily—once upon awakening and once before going to sleep. Prof
states, "The hardest part is beginning to do them and then
sustaining it." Writing the affirmations on a sheet of paper and
posting them on your bathroom mirror or inside a cupboard door

may work for you. Another option is to record them (most of us have cell phones we can use for audio recording) in your own voice and listen to them.

Here are some of the self-affirmations we found helpful:

- I can cope.
- I can make compromises in my lifestyle in order to heal.
- I can manage my pain successfully.
- I am a strong person.
- I will overcome this adversity.
- I have faith and trust in my ability to cope.
- I will successfully manage this procedure.
- I am prepared for whatever comes my way.
- I have very supportive and loving family and friends.
- I will find strength and courage to overcome the effects of this illness and its treatment.
- I am able to maintain control and respond appropriately to this situation.
- I am confident with this treatment.
- I can manage this daily life and its demands.
- I believe in myself.
- I will rest and heal as required.
- I trust my inner strengths as a person and know I am capable of managing this.
- I can depend on those close to me to help me through this difficult time.
- I will manage this experience well for my own good and for the good of all I love.
- I will survive.
- I believe I can and will transcend my illness.
- I will be a treatment success.
- I will transcend the effects of illness and treatment and enjoy each moment in life.
- I am planning for my happy and successful future.
- The tumor has been dealt with.
- I have the patience to help me through the treatment and healing process.
- I believe this storm will pass.
- I am well.
- I am healthy.

- I am healing.
- I have a healthy colon.
- My rectum/anus is healing.
- I have a wonderful partner.
- I am loved.
- I work hard to be connected to others.
- I keep communication open with important others.
- I am looking toward my future with hope.
- I am getting stronger.
- I am going to survive.
- I am going to live long.
- I will get through this.
- My optimal mental health is the key to good health.
- I feel peace, ease, freedom, and relaxation.
- I have faith in my healthcare team.
- I will do everything I can to restore my body to wellness.
- I am receiving and am grateful for many amazing and miraculous blessings.

Note: If you have a belief in God or a higher power, you may want to add some affirmations with this in mind.

****

RESOURCES:

Prof. Wolkenstein fully utilized (over 1,000 times) Belleruth Naparstek's **Health Journeys: Cancer**, Hachette Audio Series (1993). More of her meditation and guided imagery products can be found online at *healthjourneys.com/audio-library/cancer*.

For more great ideas, check out **FreeAffirmations.org** on the Internet. They have a listing for Survive Cancer Positive Affirmations—*freeaffirmations.org/survive-cancer-positive-affirmations*. This is a unique set of affirmations to help you acquire a "survive cancer" mindset.

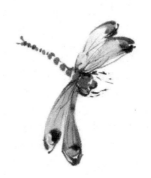

Anal Cancer Supplies List*

Angela G. Gentile

NOTE: If you're not sure, make sure you ask your doctor if you can take or use any of these, as you don't want to use anything that could cause you more harm than good.

Pick and choose what you think you would like/need, and not all items will be available in your country. Always ask your oncology team about treatments that may interfere with radiation or chemotherapy.

Tools:
- Date minder or Cancer Treatment organizer (I also used the calendar on my phone)
- Journal to write in
- Digital thermometer
- Sitz bath
- Tablet or laptop and cellular service or Wi-Fi to surf the Internet or use social media, listen to music, read, watch movies/series
- Books, magazines, movies, music
- Book of prayers
- Fan (to cool down hot, radiated skin)
- Vaginal dilators (to help prevent or reduce scarring and stenosis)
- Handheld magnifying mirror

For the bath and shower:
- Baking Soda
- Epsom salt
- Handheld shower nozzle
- Cetaphil bar soap (gentle skin care)
- Baby shampoo

- Invati Advanced Hair Loss Treatment & Thinning Hair Shampoos by Aveda (very expensive—look for alternatives!)
- Leave-in hair conditioner for dry, damaged, or thinning hair

For the body:
- Antibacterial hand sanitizer (for yourself, and keep one by the door for others who come to visit!)
- Lip balm
- Sensitive skin baby wipes
- Perineal irrigation bottle (plastic squirt bottle)
- Comfort Shield® Barrier Cream Cloths (with Dimethicone)
- Glaxal Base®—moisturizing cream
- Head scarves, wigs, or caps
- Loose-fitting skirts, dresses, pants or shorts
- Warm fuzzy socks
- Memory Foam® mattress topper (this is so comfy!)
- Extra towels and sheets (I also made small washable cotton pads from baby receiving blankets)
- Disposable or washable underpads (soaker pad) to protect the bed
- Disposable latex gloves
- Disposable latex finger cots (goes on the fingertip, for applying ointments)
- Depend® or other brand of incontinence underwear
- Disposable mesh panties (by size)
- Cotton underpants or boxers a couple sizes bigger than your usual
- Panty liners with wings (for diarrhea or wound discharge)
- Frozen or icy mitts or socks (to help prevent neuropathy)

For the mouth (for chemotherapy-induced challenges):
- Biotene® mouthwash and toothpaste
- Soft toothbrush
- Toothpaste for sensitive guns
- "Magic Mouthwash" for mouth sores (by prescription)
- Flexible straws
- Oracoat XyliMelts® for Dry Mouth

For the bottom (for radiation therapy-induced challenges and burns):

- Imodium® (loperamide, to reduce the frequency of diarrhea)
- Stool softeners/laxatives (e.g., Metamucil®, docusate sodium, Senokot-S®)
- AZO Urinary Pain Relief® tablets
- Chair pillow
- Memory Foam® and/or gel cushion
- ROHO® cushion (expensive adjustable pressure-relieving cushion)
- Donut/Ring/Invalid seat cushion
- Pain medication (prescription and non-prescription)—Examples: acetaminophen (Tylenol®), ibuprofen (Advil®), naproxen sodium (Aleve®), oxycodone hydrochloride (Oxycontin®), morphine, gabapentin (Neurontin®), CBD oil, fentanyl, hydromorphone (Dilaudid®), cortisone, ketamine. Ask about formats such as oral, IV, compounds, sprays, and patches. Numbing cream (ex, Lidocane 5%, LMX 5% Topical Anorectal Cream)
- Special pain cream compounds with lidocaine, Nifedioine, Morphine, Sucral, Mediderm®, ketamine, dimethyl sulfoxide or DMSO, gabapentin (prescription required)
- Stress balls (to help with pain or stress management)
- Flexible soft gel ice packs
- Flamazine/Silvadene (Silver Sulfadiazine 1%) (by prescription)
- Aquaphor
- Proshield® Plus (Dimethicone Ointment Skin Protectant)
- Vitamin E skin oil
- Coconut oil
- Domeboro® Soak
- Instillagel®—anesthetic antiseptic lubricant (UK)
- Desitin® Cream (zinc oxide)
- A & D® Ointment (lanolin and petrolatum) barrier cream
- Aloe Vera gel
- Vagisil®—to relieve external vaginal itching and irritation
- Polysporin® Topical Ointment—speeds healing and prevents infection
- Anusol®—hemorrhoid treatment and pain relief
- Calmoseptine® ointment—protects and helps heal skin irritations (burns/irradiated skin)

- Zum Rub® Moisturizer (includes shea butter)
- Dressings such as Non-Stick Dressings Absorbent Compress (protects) by Elastoplast®
- DermaPlast®—for treatment of minor wounds (can be found in a spray bottle format)
- Eletone® cream—nonsteroidal barrier cream, works as an emollient (by prescription only)
- Miaderm® radiation relief skin cream
- Emu soap and oil—for radiated skin
- Corn starch or Pure Cornstarch Baby Powder—to help keep area dry

For your tummy:
- Probiotics
- Antinausea medication (Ex. Metoclopramide HCL, prochlorperazine maleate) by prescription
- Gravol®
- Pepto-Bismol® for upset stomach and diarrhea relief (I used the tablets)
- Greek Yogurt (high in protein)
- Applesauce
- Clear broth
- Veggies for juicing
- Greens for drinks
- Nut butter
- Eggs
- Tuna
- Bread that is not high in fiber
- Sorbet
- Gatorade®
- Boost/Ensure (liquid nutritional supplement)
- Juven®—Therapeutic nutrition drink mix to support healing
- Ginger ale (to relieve nausea)

Other ideas:
- Peppermint essential oil (I used this to help me cope with the smell from the chemo pump—I put a little on my upper lip).
- Lavender essential oil (I used this to help me relax and sleep)
- Ear plugs (to help you sleep or give to your family

members when things get rough!)
- A bag or backpack to carry a change of clothes, paper towels, wipes, plastic bags, etc. for accidents (keep one in the car and one with you). I called mine my "Butt Bag."
- Extra towels for sitting on, especially if you are in someone else's car or home.
- Squatty Potty®—The original toilet stool.

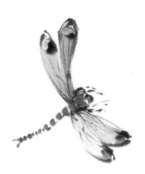

Glossary

Abdominoperineal resection (APR)
Surgery to remove the anus, the rectum, and part of the sigmoid colon through an incision made in the abdomen. The end of the intestine is attached to an opening in the surface of the abdomen and body waste is collected in a disposable bag outside of the body. This opening is called a colostomy. Lymph nodes that contain cancer may also be removed during this operation. National Cancer Institute (NCI)

Alternative medicine
A complementary and alternative medicine (CAM) therapy used in place of standard treatments.
(Office of Cancer Complementary and Alternative Medicine, *cam.cancer.gov*).

Anal cancer
Anal cancer is an uncommon type of cancer that occurs in the anal canal. The anal canal is the short tube at the end of your rectum through which stool leaves your body. (*mayoclinic.org*)

Anoscopy
A procedure that uses an anoscope (a short, hollow tube-like instrument that may have a light) to examine the anus. (Canadian Cancer Society, *info.cancer.ca*)

Biopsy
The removal of cells or tissues for examination by a pathologist. The pathologist may study the tissue under a microscope or perform other tests on the cells or tissue. There are many different types of biopsy procedures. The most common types include: (1) incisional biopsy, in which only a sample of tissue is removed; (2) excisional biopsy, in which an entire lump or suspicious area is removed; and (3) needle biopsy, in which a sample of tissue or fluid is removed

with a needle. When a wide needle is used, the procedure is called a core biopsy. When a thin needle is used, the procedure is called a fine-needle aspiration biopsy. NCI

Brachytherapy
A type of radiation therapy in which radioactive material sealed in needles, seeds, wires, or catheters is place directly into or near a tumor. Also called implant radiation therapy, internal radiation therapy, and radiation brachytherapy. NCI

Cancerversary
Like a cancer experience, the cancerversary is unique. It is a milestone defined by the person. It might be the day of cancer diagnosis. It might be the last day of treatment. It might be the day the doctor gave the all-clear (cancer-free news). It may be several important dates that occur throughout someone's cancer journey. (National Coalition for Cancer Survivorship, *canceradvocacy.org*)

Chemo brain
A common term used by cancer survivors to describe thinking and memory problems that can occur after cancer treatment. Chemo brain can also be called chemo fog, chemotherapy-related cognitive impairment or cognitive dysfunction.
(Mayo Clinic, *mayoclinic.org*)

Chemoradiation
Treatment that combines chemotherapy with radiation therapy. Also called chemoradiotherapy. NCI

Chemotherapy
Treatment that uses drugs to stop the growth of cancer cells, either by killing the cells or by stopping them from dividing. NCI

Colonoscopy
Examination of the inside of the colon using a colonoscope, inserted into the rectum. A colonoscope is a thin, tube-like instrument with a light and a lens for viewing. It may also have a tool to remove tissue to be checked under a microscope for signs of disease. NCI

Colorectal surgeon
A general surgeon who has had further training and is an expert in the diagnosis and treatment of benign and malignant disease of the colon, rectum and anus. (MedicineNet, *medicinenet.com*)

Complementary and alternative medicine (CAM)
Any medical system, practice, or product that is not thought of as standard care. (Office of Cancer Complementary and Alternative Medicine, *cam.cancer.gov*)

Complementary medicine
A CAM therapy used along with standard medicine. (Office of Cancer Complementary and Alternative Medicine, *cam.cancer.gov*)

CT scan
A procedure that uses a computer linked to an x-ray machine to make a series of detailed pictures of areas inside the body. The pictures are taken from different angles and areas and used to create three-dimensional (3-D) views of tissues and organs. A dye may be injected into a vein or swallowed to help the tissues and organs show up more clearly. A CT scan may be used to help diagnosis disease, plan treatment, or find out how well treatment is working. Also called CAT scan, computed tomography scan, computerized axial tomography scan, and computerized tomography. NCI

Depend®
A brand of absorbent, disposable underwear for adults. (*depend.com*)

Digital Rectal Examination (DRE)
An examination in which a doctor inserts a lubricated, gloved finger into the rectum to feel for abnormalities. NCI

Endoscopy
A procedure that uses an endoscope to examine the inside of the body. An endoscope is a thin, tube-like instrument with a light and a lens for viewing. It may also have a tool to remove tissue to be checked under a microscope for signs of disease. NCI

Fluorouracil
Also known as 5-FU. Fluorouracil is the generic name for a chemotherapy drug. Xeloda is the oral pill form.

Gastroenterologist
A doctor who has special training in diagnosing and treating disorders of the digestive system. NCI

Gastrointestinal tract
The stomach and intestines. The gastrointestinal tract is part of the digestive system, which also includes the salivary glands, mouth, esophagus, liver, pancreas, gallbladder, and rectum. NCI

Human papillomavirus (HPV)
A type of virus that can cause abnormal tissue growth (for example, genital and anal warts) and other changes to cells. Infections for a long time with certain types of HPV can cause cervical cancer. HPV may also play a role in some other types of cancer, such as anal, vaginal, penile, and oropharyngeal cancers. NCI

Immunotherapy
A type of therapy that uses substances to stimulate or suppress the immune system to help the body fight cancer, infection, and other diseases. Some types of immunotherapy only target certain cells of the immune system. Others affect the immune system in a general way. Types of immunotherapy include cytokines, vaccines, bacillus Calmette-Guerin (BCG), and some monoclonal antibodies. NCI

Integrative medicine
An approach that combines treatments from conventional medicine and CAM for which there is some high-quality evidence of safety and effectiveness. (Office of Cancer Complementary and Alternative Medicine, *cam.cancer.gov*)

Late effects
A late effect is a side effect that occurs months or years after cancer treatment. Many people who have received treatment for cancer have a risk of developing long-term side effects. In fact, evaluating and treating late effects is an important part of survivorship care. (*cancer.net*)

Lymphatic system
The group of tissues and organs that produce and store cells that fight infection and diseases. The lymphatic system includes the adenoids, tonsils, spleen, thymus, lymph nodes, lymph vessels, and bone marrow. Also called the lymph system. (Canadian Cancer Society, *info.cancer.ca*)

Lymph node
A small bean-shaped mass of lymphatic tissue along lymph vessels (tubes through which lymph fluid travels in the body). Lymph nodes store lymphocytes (a type of white blood cell that fights germs, foreign substances, or cancer cells) and filters bacteria and foreign substances (including cancer cells) from lymph fluid. (Canadian Cancer Society, *info.cancer.ca*)

Magnetic resonance imaging (MRI)
A procedure in which radio waves and a powerful magnet linked to a computer are used to create detailed pictures of areas inside the body. These pictures can show the difference between normal and diseased tissue. MRI makes better images of organs and soft tissue than other scanning techniques, such as computed tomography (CT) or x-ray. MRI is especially useful for imaging the brain, the spine, the soft tissue of joints, and the inside of bones. Also called NMRI, and nuclear magnetic resonance imaging. NCI

Malignant
Another word for cancerous.

Metastasis
The spread of cancer cells from the place where they first formed to another part of the body. In metastasis, cancer cells break away from the original (primary) tumor, travel through the blood or lymph system, and form a new tumor in other organs or tissues of the body. The new, metastatic tumor is the same type of cancer as the primary tumor. For example, if breast cancer spreads to the lung, the cancer cells in the lung are breast cancer cells, not lung cancer cells. The plural form of metastasis is metastases. NCI

Mitomycin
The generic name for a chemotherapy drug. Also known as Mitomycin-C.

Mouth sores
Cancer-related mouth sores form on the inside lining of your mouth or on your lips. The mouth sores appear burn-like and can be painful, making it difficult to eat, talk, swallow, and breathe. Sores can appear on any of the soft tissues of your lips or your mouth, including the gums, tongue, and roof or floor of the mouth. Sores can also extend into the tube (esophagus) that carries food to your stomach. (*mayoclinic.org*)

Neutropenia
A condition in which there is a lower than normal number of neutrophils (a type of white blood cell) in the blood. NCI

Nigro Protocol
Developed in the 1970s, this anal cancer treatment was developed by Dr. Norman Nigro. His protocol of 3,000 rads of external beam radiation, a five-day infusion of 5-flourouracil, and a single injection of Mitomycin-C became known as the "Nigro Protocol" and later signified a major advancement in the treatment of anal cancer, and in oncology in general. Further refinements would lead to combined chemotherapy and radiation therapy as the primary treatment for anal carcinoma with most patients successfully treated without surgery (Osborne et. al, 2014).

No evidence of disease (NED)
If a patient is in partial remission, it may mean s/he can take a break from treatment as long as the cancer doesn't begin to grow again. Complete remission means that tests, physical exams, and scans show that all signs of cancer are gone. Some doctors also refer to complete remission as "no evidence of disease."
(WebMD, *webmd.com*)

Oncologist
A doctor who has special training in diagnosing and treating cancer. Some oncologists specialize in a particular type of cancer treatment. For example, a radiation oncologist specializes in treating cancer with radiation. A medical oncologist prescribes chemotherapy. NCI

Oncology
A branch of medicine that specializes in the diagnosis and treatment of cancer. It includes medical oncology (the use of chemotherapy, hormone therapy, and other drugs to treat cancer), radiation oncology (the use of radiation therapy to treat cancer), and surgical oncology (the use of surgery and other procedures to treat cancer). NCI

PET scan
Also called positron emission tomography scan. A procedure in which a small amount of radioactive glucose (sugar) is injected into a vein, and a scanner is used to make detailed, computerized pictures of areas inside the body where the glucose is taken up. Because cancer cells often take up more glucose than normal cells, the pictures can be used to find cancer cells in the body. NCI

Pelvic floor physiotherapy/physical therapy
Pelvic floor physical therapy involves the pelvic floor muscle group, which is responsible for a variety of functions. These muscles support the pelvic organs, assist in bowel and bladder control, and contribute to sexual arousal and orgasm. A person may be referred to pelvic floor physical therapy to treat incontinence, difficulty with urination or bowel movements, constipation, chronic pelvic pain, and painful intercourse. (*issm.info*)

Pelvic Radiation Disease (PRD)
Any brief or long-lasting problems which can be anything from very mild to very severe, arising in normal, noncancerous tissues and which start as a result of radiotherapy to a tumor in the pelvis. People who develop new symptoms affecting the bowel, urinary tract, sex organs, bones, or skin during or after radiotherapy may have PRD.
(Pelvic Radiation Disease Association, *prda.org.uk*)

Perianal
Pertaining to the area around the anus.

Peripherally inserted central catheter (PICC)
A long thin soft tube is inserted in the superior vena cava vein by a medical team. It is placed in the arm, near or just above the bend in the elbow. This device allows the medical team to administer

medication, provide chemotherapy/intravenous fluids/blood transfusions, and it also allows for easy access to blood samples. It remains in the arm for the duration of treatment. (Health Sciences Centre, Winnipeg)

Polyp
A small clump of cells that grow inside your body. Some are benign (noncancerous), others can turn into cancer.

Port or implanted central vascular access device (CVAD)
This small metal device is placed under the skin in the upper chest area. It is attached to a long soft tube that is inserted into a large vein for quick and easy access. It can be used for giving medication, fluids, nutrition, chemotherapy treatments, and/or blood transfusions. It is also used for taking blood samples. It is kept in for the duration of treatment. (Health Sciences Centre, Winnipeg).

Proctoscope
A proctoscope is an examination of the anal cavity, rectum and sigmoid colon by means of a proctoscopy (a medical procedure to examine the anal cavity, rectum, or sigmoid colon using a proctoscope).

Proctosigmoidoscopy
A combined proctoscopy and sigmoidoscopy.
(*See "Sigmoidoscopy."*)

Prognosis
The likely outcome or course of a disease; the chance of recovery or recurrence. NCI

Radiation burns
Radiation therapy uses high-energy radiation or radioactive substances to shrink or kill cancerous cells. When radiation passes through the skin, the skin cells in the treatment area may become damaged. After frequent radiation treatments, skin cells often do not have enough time to repair and regenerate between treatments. Radiation therapy may cause the exposed skin to peel off more quickly than it can grow back, causing sores or ulcers. While these wounds may look and feel like burns, the term is a misnomer, since the treatment does not actually burn the skin. For it to heal, the skin

needs time to regenerate, a process that may take two to four weeks for mild reactions, or several months or more for serious injuries. In the interim, various integrative therapies may be used to soothe the itching and pain that often results. Acute skin reactions, ranging from a slight rash to severe ulcerated or blistered skin, are common side effects of radiation treatment. An estimated 85 percent of patients who undergo radiation therapy experience moderate to severe skin reactions, according to *Current Oncology,* a peer-reviewed medical journal. Acute reactions to radiation treatments may lead to itchiness, pain, and reduced quality of life. (*cancercenter.com*)

Radiation therapy (RT) or Radiotherapy
The use of high-energy radiation from x-rays, gamma rays, neutrons, protons, and other sources to kill cancer cells and shrink tumors. Radiation may come from a machine outside the body (external-beam radiation therapy), or it may come from radioactive material placed in the body near cancer cells (internal radiation therapy or brachytherapy). Systemic radiation therapy uses a radioactive substance, such as a radio-labeled monoclonal antibody, that travels in the blood to tissues throughout the body. Also called irradiation. NCI

Sigmoidoscopy
Examination of the lower colon using a sigmoidoscope, inserted into the rectum. A sigmoidoscope is a thin, tube-like instrument with a light and a lens for viewing. It may also have a tool to remove tissue to be checked under a microscope for signs of disease. Also called proctosigmoidoscopy. NCI

Squamous cell carcinoma
Cancer that begins in squamous cells. Squamous cells are thin, flat cells that look like fish scales, and are found in the tissue that forms the surface of the skin, the lining of the hollow organs of the body, and the lining of the respiratory and digestive tracts. Most cancers of the anus, cervix, head and neck, and vagina are squamous cell carcinomas. Also called epidermoid carcinoma. NCI

Staging
Performing exams and tests to learn the extent of the cancer within the body, especially whether the disease has spread from where it

first formed to other parts of the body. It is important to know the stage of the disease in order to plan the best treatment. There are four cancer stages: 1–4 (also written as I–IV). Sometimes letters such as "a" or "b" are added to provide more detail. NCI

Survivor
A cancer survivor is one who remains alive and continues to function during and after overcoming a serious hardship or life-threatening disease. In cancer, a person is considered to be a survivor from the time of diagnosis until the end of life. NCI

Thriver
The Human Papillomavirus (HPV) and Anal Cancer Foundation's term for cancer survivor. (*analcancerfoundation.org*)

Tumor
An abnormal mass of tissue that results when cells divide more than they should or do not die when they should. Tumors may be benign (no cancer) or malignant (cancer). Also called neoplasm. NCI

White blood cells
White blood cells protect the body against infection. Some types of white blood cells include lymphocytes, monocytes, and eosinophils. Each type of white blood cell plays a different role in protecting the body. The numbers of each type of white blood cells give important information about the immune system. Too many or too few of the different types of white blood cells can help identify an infection, an allergic or toxic reaction to medicines or chemicals, and many conditions, such as leukemia. (WebMD, *webmd.com*)

****

REFERENCES:

National Cancer Institute (NCI) (*cancer.gov*)

Osborne, M. C., Maykel, J. & Steele, S. R. (2014). Anal Squamous Cell Carcinoma: An Evolution In Disease and Management. *World Journal of Gastroenterology*, Sep 28: 20 (36), 13052-13059. Retrieved 04 Feb 2018. (*ncbi.nlm.nih.gov*)

Resources

FOR FURTHER READING:

Draeger, Bonnie E. (2012). *When Cancer Strikes a Friend: What to Say, What to Do, and How to Help*. USA: Skyhorse Publishing.

Lemole, G. M., Mehta, P. K. And McKee, D. L. (2015). *After Cancer Care: The definitive self-care guide to getting and staying well for patients after cancer*. USA: Rodale.

Longabaugh, Michele (2012). *If You're Not Laughing, You're Dying: The dawning of hope from the shadows of darkness...blogging through stage 4 anal cancer*. Kindle edition eBook.

Mayhew, Theresa (2010). *Kicking Cancer in the Butt*. USA: Createspace.

Woolard, Robbi (2016). *Brown Ribbon: A Personal Journey Through Anal Cancer and the Adventure it Entailed* (2016). Kindle edition eBook.

Kushner, Harold S. (2004). *When Bad Things Happen to Good People*. USA: Anchor Books.

ONLINE RESOURCES:

American Cancer Society (*cancer.org*)

American Cancer Society Cancer Action Network (*acscan.org*)

Canadian Cancer Society (*cancer.ca*)

Centers for Disease Control and Prevention (*cdc.gov*)

ChemoCare (*chemocare.com*)

Cochrane (*cochrane.org*)

The Farrah Fawcett Foundation
(*thefarrahfawcettfoundation.org*)

The HPV and Anal Cancer Foundation
(*analcancerfoundation.org*)

The HPV and Anal Cancer Foundation's Peer to Peer Program
(*analcancerfoundation.org/find-support/patientsupport/connect -with-a-peer/*)

Mayo Clinic (*mayoclinic.org*)

National Cancer Institute (*cancer.gov*)

National Comprehensive Cancer Network Guidelines for Anal Carcinoma (Login required)
(*nccn.org/professionals/physician_gls/PDF/anal.pdf*)

National Institutes of Health (*nih.gov*)

Pelvic Radiation Disease Association in the UK
(*prda.org.uk*)

PubMed (*ncbi.nlm.nih.gov/pubmed/*)

Quackwatch (*quackwatch.org*)

PERSONAL BLOGS AND WEBSITES:

Anal About Cancer by Laura Zick-Mauzy
(*analaboutcancer.com*)

Anal Cancer Help (*analcancerhelp.info*)

Anal Cancer It's a Pain in the Butt Literally
(*facebook.com/AnalCancerRibbonPage/*)

Anal Cancer is Really Shtty by Susan Anderson Molenda
(*facebook.com/analcancerisreallyshtty/* and
analcancerisreallyshitty.com)

Anal_Cancer Support Facebook Group
(*www.facebook.com/groups/analcancersupport/*)

Blog for a Cure (*blogforacure.com*)

Butt Support—Joy Anderson Facebook Page
(*facebook.com/groups/246261082228812/*)

Join Jodi's Journey—CaringBridge
(*caringbridge.org/visit/joinjodisjourney*)

Sharie's Blog—Anal Cancer: Anus Funny as You Think
(*anusfunnyasyouthink.com*)

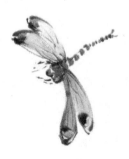

Contributor Bios

Joy Anderson is a soon-to-be 62-year-old Army veteran, retired wallpaper hanger, grandmother of five, and festival director for Earth Spirit People. She lives in a small town on a five-acre farm in Texas with her boyfriend of 17 years and his son. She rates the "crazy cat lady" moniker, as at this time she has 20 indoor/outdoor cats. She also has a service dog, a blue and gold macaw, several chickens, and a couple of goats. She loves camping, arts and crafts, swimming, and plans to get back into light hiking. She is also a member of a military women's art group.

Maria L. Barr was born in Massachusetts and grew up in Montville, Connecticut. She has four siblings. Although she and her sister are two years apart, people thought they were twins. She graduated high school in 1987 and has a Bachelor's degree in Business Administration. She has three adult children (including twins!) and lives with her significant other in Florida. She enjoys music and the outdoors. Maria has enjoyed a lifelong passion for natural healing and overall well-being support (meditation, etc.) and is well-versed in the areas of spiritual quests. She is also a big fan of the Science Channel.

Sharon Basic was born in London, Ontario. She is the youngest of five children. She obtained her BA from the University of Western Ontario and her teaching degree from London Teacher's College. For 31 years she taught for the London Board of Education, which has now been renamed the Thames Valley District School Board. Fourteen of those years were in regular primary classes and 17 years in primary Special Education classes. She was married to her husband Ferdo for 31 years before his death from colorectal cancer. She lives with her goldendoodle Baylee on a small farm on the outskirts of London, Ontario, Canada.

Peggy Belton grew up living in the Midwest as the daughter of self-employed baby-boomers. It was there that she learned about hard work and integrity and tapped into her passion for medical science. She began her professional years as a Radiologic Technologist. Years later, she returned to school and obtained her

BA in Management of Health Services from Ottawa University. She presently works as an Area Vice President for a national wound care management company. Peggy lives in Iowa with her husband Guy and their three shedding machines (also known as cats). As a Christian couple, Peggy and Guy "stepped over the faith line" in 2016. She enjoys quilting, crafting, and home improvements in her free time and is hopeful that Samantha, Levi, Sydney, or Drew will bless her with a grandchild one day.

Jodi Canaday Green grew up in West Virginia but relocated to Nashville, Tennessee, in 1994 to attend Belmont University. She graduated from Belmont in 1997 with a BS and then received her master's degree in 2004 from Trevecca Nazarene University. In 2014 she received her Doctorate from Union University. Currently, she is a middle school principal in Gallatin, Tennessee. Jodi is married to Golden. They have four children, Hunter, Alexi, Emma Claire, and Jonas, and one granddaughter, Willow Ann. She attends church at Goodlettsville Church of the Nazarene and is a committee member for the local Relay For Life. Jodi enjoys reading, traveling, the beach, and family time.

Marshall Carter-Tripp is a retired political science professor, diplomat, and museum director. She experienced medical care in Nigeria, Panama, Belgium, Spain, Portugal, and Argentina as well as the US. One difference to note: in several of those, the patient was given the scan, mammogram, or xray reports to keep, and it was her decision and responsibility to maintain them and share with other doctors! Marshall has co-authored two political science textbooks and numerous articles, and written travel articles about Spain and Argentina, which were published in the local press. She is currently active in the regional cancer foundation's programs.

Michael DeHart is a social entrepreneur, rock climber, and proud adoptive father of two Kenyan sons. He has a Bachelor's degree in mathematics from San Francisco State University and an Executive MBA from Golden Gate University. He is the Managing Partner at Cognition Market Research and CEO/Founder of East African Social Ventures—a social enterprise organization dedicated to sustainable job creation for African citizens. He lives in Sacramento, California, for now, and will be splitting time between California and Kenya after he's finished with his cancer treatments.

Joana Dougherty McGee, MA, is a many-hat-wearing bilingual (Spanish) educator and counselor, who works with children who have cancer and with their families. She is also a specialist in child-loss bereavement. Disabled from the last bout with cancer, she now does most of her work online. Other professional endeavors include decades of public high school teaching (satisfying for a high school dropout!), singing, beading, and writing. She has always championed "the underdog," and works with her community as much as possible, giving workshops and facilitating family and bereavement groups. She lives in the redwood and oak-studded coastal forests of northern California with her husband, four dogs, and three parrots. Soon, she will be relocating permanently to Europe.

Susan (Sue) Anderson Molenda has been acting and writing since middle school. She studied fine art and theatre at Augustana College, Illinois, and Media Arts and Animation through the Art Institute of Pittsburgh, and a few other places, never quite finding the impetus to complete a degree before cancer set in, possibly long before her diagnosis in 2010. She is a freelance actor, playwright, and screenwriter. She is also a freelance portrait artist who works in many media. Sue has three daughters, one son, and a very attentive rabbit. All share her affinity for the arts (the rabbit loves good music) and for healthy, vegan foods. Check out her blog and get ready to order her first memoir book at *analcancerisreallyshitty.com.*

Calvin Nokes is a cancer survivor and a partner in a long-term committed relationship of 24 years. He attended high school in Virginia decades ago and in 2010 graduated with an Associate's Degree in Health Care Administration from the University of Phoenix. He enjoys soap opera, home cooking, and time with his cats. Calvin is committed to lobbying for Cancer research funding and raising awareness of anal cancer.

Sheila Roy was born in Winnipeg, Manitoba. She's been married for 32 years and has two adult children. She is a diagnostic X-ray technologist with 30 years of experience, working full-time in a pain management clinic at Health Sciences Centre in Winnipeg. She enjoys spending time at her cottage with her husband. Some of her favorite times are spent with her spirited dog Olive, her "golden child."

Virginia Davis Wilson was born in raised in Toronto, Ontario. She raised three children, was married for 30 years, and divorced in 1996. She is presently working as a personal support worker (PSW). Reading and writing have always been her passion. She is currently living in cottage country north of Toronto.

Sharie Vance is a native Texan, mother of four, and a grandmother of seven. She's also an anal cancer survivor. During her treatment, she was a non-traditional graduate student. Sharie now holds an MFA in documentary film production from the University of North Texas. In addition to making documentary films, she teaches video production full-time at a local community college, journals extensively, occasionally writes poetry, paints, and plays the harmonica whenever she gets the chance. Sharie is a newlywed. She and her husband, Don, share a townhome in Dallas, Texas, with her father, only son, and youngest daughter.

Alan S. Wolkenstein, MSW, ACSW, is a retired Clinical Professor of Family Medicine at the University of Wisconsin School of Medicine and Public Health. For over 30 years, he taught primary care residents the biopsychosocial model of health care, humanism in medicine, and a perspective that residents and all learners need to be reflective in their work, enhance their self-awareness (mindfulness), and develop psychological depth (be "in the moment" with sick persons). "Prof" has lived with and through prostate cancer and has consulted with over 100 men and their families in helping them choose the pathway of their lives. He believes we all have deep inner voices of wisdom and clarity that can help us in the challenging and difficult circumstances of cancer. Sometimes, we need a guide or mentor to facilitate our hearing these voices.

Laura Zick-Mauzy was born in Fairmont, West Virginia. She has a Bachelor's degree in clinical laboratory science and works part-time as a medical laboratory scientist at a small rural hospital. When she isn't working, she enjoys writing, blogging, photography, painting, and traveling. Nothing makes her happier, though, than family—spending time with her two adult sons, four bonus children (she won't subscribe to the term "step-children"), and their twelve grand and two great-grand kids. Today, Laura, her husband Paul, and their three little dogs reside in Parsons, West Virginia. Her best-selling memoir about her cancer journey hasn't yet been published <<smiling>>; however, if you'd like to know more about when that book will be released, please visit her blog at *analaboutcancer.com*.

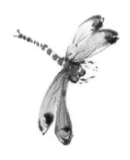

The Dragonfly Story

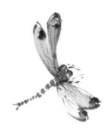 *In the bottom of an old pond lived some grubs who could not understand why none of their group ever came back after crawling up the lily stems to the top of the water. They promised each other that the next one who was called to make the upward climb would return and tell what had happened to him. Soon one of them felt an urgent impulse to seek the surface; he rested himself on the top of a lily pad and went through a glorious transformation which made him a dragonfly with beautiful wings. In vain he tried to keep his promise. Flying back and forth over the pond, he peered down at his friends below. Then he realized that even if they could see him they would not recognize such a radiant creature as one of their number.*

The fact that our friends cannot see us or talk with us after the transformation which we call death is no proof that we cease to exist.

−Rev. Walter Dudley Cavert

REFERENCE:

Cavert, W. D. (1944). *Remember Now . . . Daily Devotionals for Young People*. USA: Festival (Original source: Albert W. Palmer, The New Christian Epic, Pilgrim Press, 1928).

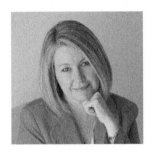

About the Author

Editor and major contributor Angela G. Gentile was born in Toronto, Ontario, and attended university in Winnipeg, Manitoba. She is a registered social worker and obtained her B.S.W. and M.S.W. at the University of Manitoba. Angela, a Specialist in Aging, is employed as a Geriatric Mental Health Clinician. She is married to Agapito (a.k.a. Cupp) and has two adult children, Lorenzo and Simone. She enjoys writing, reading, and traveling, and considers herself a realistic optimist. Additionally, she has a passion for sharing her knowledge of complementary medicine and exploring the depths of spirituality. She resides in Winnipeg with her husband, daughter, and two dogs.

For more information: www.AngelaGGentile.com

INDEX

Glossary entries in **bold**. Figures in ***bold italics***.

F
faith in a higher power, 108, 143, 144, 147, 152, 186, 194, 197, 199, 201, 205, 276
fatigue, 10, 11, 22, 57, 98, 99, 122, 146, 148, 182
Farrah Fawcett, iii, 4, 5, 191, 223, 224, 228
Farrah Fawcett Foundation, 4, 16, 229, 230, 272
fear:
    cancer, 17, 23-24, 65, 67, 73, 115-117, 119-121, 129-130, 137-140, 142, 144, 150, 151, 160, 165, 168, 179, 181-182, 185-186, 196, 199, 204, 207-208, 210
    embarrassment, 46, 51
    failure, 73, 82, 204
    losing hair, 60
    recurrence, 14-15, 61, 123, 246
    stigma, 127
    strategies to deal with, 251-253
fever, 33, 58
financial issues, 17, 20, 21, 24, 72, 81, 129, 195, 237
fistula, 5, 98
fissure, 5
5-FU. *See* fluorouracil.
fluorouracil, 8, 56, 72, 90, 154, **264**
FODMAP, 96
follow-up, 8, 14, 15, 31, 45, 60, 123
Frankl, Viktor, 190
Frazzoni, L., 109
Friedman, H., 190
frustration, 24, 98, 117, 155
fundraising, iii, 20, 21, 163, 226, 228, 234, 277
future after cancer, 68, 83, 147, 159, 164,176, 187, 229, 233, 252, 253

G
gastroenterologist, 94, 95, 130, **264**
gastrointestinal tract, 2, 13, 51, 93-95, **264**
genital:
    warts, 6, 264
    burns, 9
Ghoshal, S., 22, 38
Greaves, Lynda Sie, 141-152

Green, Jodie Canaday, 111-118, 247, 276
grief, 23-25, 37, 38, 57, 61, 75, 141, 143, 151, 160, 176, 184, 200, 224, 249
groin, 4, 9, 12, 42, 45
Gross, C. P., 159, 172
guilt, 24, 120, 160
gynecologist, 6, 7, 30, 35, 192

H
Haboubi, N. Y., 94, 96, 109
Hauer-Jensen, M., 95, 96, 109
hair loss, 11, 17, 44, 57, 60, 91, 122, 256
helpless, 25, 57, 146, 147, 180, 196, 205
hemorrhoids, 5, 7, 41, 45, 46, 56, 130, 192, 203, 215, 223, 240, 257
herbs, 12, 32, 161, 166, 167, 170, 171
Hollen, Carol Anne, iv, 95
human immunodeficiency virus (HIV), 6, 7, 153, 156, 221-224, 226
human papillomavirus (HPV), 2, 4, 6, 7, 15, 52, 192-194, 197, 229, 240, **264**
HPV and Anal Cancer Foundation, The, iii, 2, 16, 229, 230, 270, 272
HPV vaccine, iii, 7, 194, 197, 227
hyperbaric oxygen therapy, 95

I
immune system, 6, 10, 104, 168, 186, 221, 224, **264**, 270
immunotherapy, 13, 20, 160, 246, **264**
incontinence. *See* bladder control *and* bowel control.
infections, 2, 6, 7, 10, 33, 58, 98, 105, 106, 133, 153, 168, 240, 257, 264, 265, 270
infertility, 98
insurance, 20, 21, 24, 45, 129, 130, 132, 194, 195, 217, 224, 245
intimacy. *See* sexuality.
integrative medicine, 13, 14, 19, 159, 167, 171, **264,** 269

287

Made in the USA
Columbia, SC
09 May 2023

16272616R00166